Coffee or CHEMO

EDINA ATKINSON

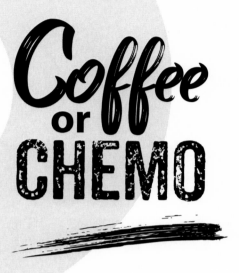

First published in Great Britain as a softback original in 2023

Copyright © Edina Atkinson

Design, typesetting and publishing by UK Book Publishing

www.ukbookpublishing.com

ISBN: 978-1-915338-72-3

Disclaimer

I have endeavoured to recreate events, locales and conversations from my own memories of them. Some names and identifying details have been changed to protect the privacy of individuals.

This book is not intended as a substitute for the medical advice of doctors. The reader should consult a doctor in matters relating to his/her health and particularly with respect to any symptoms that may require diagnosis or medical attention.

Although the author and publisher have made every effort to ensure that the information in this book was correct at press time, the author and the publisher do not assume and hereby disclaim any liability to any party for any loss, damage or disruption caused by errors or omissions, whether such errors or omissions result from negligence, accident, or any other cause.

Dedicated to all those unique individuals that I love…
and yes, you know who you are.

Contents

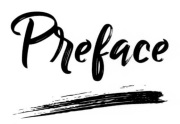

Preface

What you're about to read will sometimes fascinate, astound you and at times repulse and sicken you but stick with it because it may be very enlightening and could possibly change your life.

Coffee or Chemo will make some startling and heretical suggestions about what it really means to recover from cancer or a cancer diagnosis. The book will take you through my own personal journey of recovery and the unconventional ways of achieving a quality of healing that may be seen by some as pure quackery. However, I do advise that time is taken to read and absorb what has been written and to do your own independent research on each and every suggestion I make. I also urge you to take the time to study the real implications of conventional treatments and not to simply take the doctor's 'say-so'. The internet is a great source of instant information that in past times took years to research in a library but please be mindful the information is backed by bona fide researchers. The book's intention is to challenge all assumptions and beliefs regarding conventional medicine and healing. This book also captures my own personal beliefs and they may not match your beliefs. So it is not my intention to brainwash or coerce you into this particular set of beliefs about recovery. I looked up the word 'therapy' and its definition reads like this; "curing, healing or an activity that makes you feels happy or that helps you to deal with your problems". Tack the word chemo or radio to the front of that definition and see if it fits the interpretation? Hopefully by changing beliefs, the unnecessary physical pain of 'therapy' may be avoided. As awareness expands, it may help dispel the fear and misguided loyalty that often clouds judgement when making treatment/healing choices. Coffee or Chemo invites you to explore all treatment/healing methods that will give the very best chance for personal recovery.

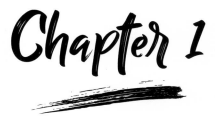

THE DREADED DIAGNOSIS

The scary truth is that I had possibly lived in almost constant fear and anxiety even before the bleak diagnosis of breast cancer but never realised it at the time. I had been scared most of my life, scared of living, afraid of dying, fearful of speaking my truth and standing up for my self, scared of making mistakes, even more fearful of the mistakes I'd already made but ultimately scared to be me. The initial diagnosis now gave me a real reason to be scared after all. Hearing the word cancer being applied to me felt like I'd been shot in the heart. I could feel the blood draining from my once healthy body which was also becoming sticky and clammy with silent hysteria. But I also intuitively knew that cancer has been marketed so cleverly that even the most well informed person would recoil in horror and possibly collapse in a heap when receiving a positive cancer diagnosis. I felt betrayed, ultimately betrayed that my body had let me down and allowed cancer to have the final blow. The word cancer is such a negative word that it's almost in alliance with the declaration of war. So just like a war the battle usually commences and nothing is ever the same again. Just like the terrain where the battle is fought I knew my body's terrain would never be the same again if I accepted the conventional treatment. But underneath the initial devastation I also had to accept this diagnosis could be a true reflection of my complete inner turmoil as to how I'd been living my life for the past 52 years.

The year leading up to the diagnosis had been fraught with personal problems regarding relationships, financial and work related issues. I'd lived on a knife edge regarding most things and I almost never felt I could entirely relax and be my true self as I 'white knuckled' myself through life. The need to present a perfect me was almost like a compulsion as I had felt inferior for most of my life. From childhood I had stuttered so badly that I had appeared dumb and that greatly reduced my confidence. I also wet the bed until I was almost seven years old. All these things had greatly diminished any ability to naturally overcome simple life issues. Bullying was a huge problem when I started secondary school and that occasionally followed me on into the workplace. My mother often used to say it was jealously but that was not much consolation when having to deal with scary bullying people on a regular basis.

My partner at the time of diagnosis took part in pharmaceutical clinical trials for financial reasons. He often lied about what he was doing, possibly in a clumsy effort to protect my feelings but more than likely to protect himself from the haranguing I would give him when I found him out. I cared about him but the devastation I felt that he could prostitute his body for pharmaceutical industry profits was beyond my comprehension. It also felt like a complete betrayal when he knew how I felt about the pharmaceutical industry and what I believed about its mafia type intentions at that time. Even before my diagnosis I knew most medication has serious side effects that could last for years and ultimately kill people in the end. I became angry and ashamed with myself for having feelings for a man that had to supplement his income from this kind of practice as he appeared to be very traditional and sensible on the surface. He would attempt to justify his participation in clinical trials with statements like he was helping society with the future development of drugs. But evidence is constantly showing clinical trials are indeed 'deeply flawed with the suppression of unfavourable results, poor regulation, diseases invented purely for profit, swollen marketing budgets, doctors and academics on the pay roll of pill manufacturers' (Ben Goldacre) But I had to accept that not everyone has the intellectual capacity to read and evaluate medical journal data to understand why unfavourable data results go missing.

Before that relationship, I had endured a emotionally abusive liaison with a covert practising alcoholic. Looking back this was like living a 'car crash' everyday. I knew the stress and anxiety was taxing my adrenal glands to such an extent that internally my body must have been breaking down. I felt like dying because

I felt so hopeless and I believe today that my body assisted that thought by producing the actual symptoms of cancer. I had a failed marriage, a daughter who I felt I had ultimately failed and a current capacity for financial ruin. At times it did seem easier to die than continue to live in such emotional pain and futility. Harbouring feelings of resentment must be the top offender for inducing symptoms of cancer and I sure as hell had a lot of resentments. My number one resentment was against myself for making so many stupid mistakes especially around my choice of a romantic partner after my marriage broke up.

Financially, I was against the wire and carried a real poverty stricken mind set. But to be honest this mind set had nearly always accompanied me in good times and bad. I was self employed and had run an exporting business that was fashionable and lucrative for a few years. When sales began to dwindle, I did whatever work I could find from sales, promotion, marketing and professional speaking to cleaning other people's homes and offices. I managed to secure a temporary contract with an estate agent which I really enjoyed but certain personality conflicts made it very difficult to continue working there so I was forced to leave simply to protect my well being. The feelings of rejection weighed heavily and so coupled with yet another failure only added to my distress. Looking back I now see myself as possibly subconsciously creating these situations. Maybe it reinforced my victim like mentality that enabled me to throw up my hands in despair and claim nothing ever works out for me.

However, an amazing marketing contract soon came my way and this stretched my capabilities into a totally different sphere. I always had the tenacity to have another go at whatever came my way so I grasped this opportunity with both hands. The owner of this company was a wealthy and attractive man but he was hard to engage with on his company's goals and aims for the future of his business. I'm still not sure why he even suggested I took on this role in his company. He appeared to respect my recommendations as his marketing manager, however; professional boundaries were crossed which then made it embarrassing to continue working together. He had given me some very contradictory messages and I believe I was too naive and probably too dazzled to understand his real motives for some of his seemingly innocent gestures at the time. So the contract really finished before I had chance to prove what I could actually do for this company. I spent several weeks replaying in my mind how I could have done it differently but looking back I don't think it would have made much difference at all. The man may have been considered player, just like some of the other men had been in my life. It appeared that I had an almost magnetic draw to these kinds of personalities. Feeling insecure always reinforced my sense of powerlessness and helplessness. This sense of powerlessness also stopped me from seeing reality and almost kept me in a fairytale fantasy.

In the meantime, I had been doing some voluntary work for a homeless charity based in my home city for about six months. This placated my misguided desire to give back to others who were less fortunate than me. Also hoping that voluntary work could pull me out of my pit of self destruction. This organisation then offered a paid part time temporary contract as a support worker. I jumped at the chance and again this role stretched me into yet another dimension as I found the job incredibly rewarding. But also quite harrowing at times witnessing the various mental health issues. Fortunately my co-workers were kind, humorous and supportive which really boosted my sense of well being as well keeping me grounded when things got occasionally tough. I became mindful that the job could be a quick burn out for many people due to the nature of some of the desperate cases the organisation took on. But along with burnout I became aware that I also identified with some of the mental health issues the organisation's clients suffered from. The only difference at times is that theirs had become official and public; mine had not.

It was during this particular uneventful but stressful time I decided to visit my GP because my left breast around the areola looked slightly retracted. I had a vague notion it might be something sinister but I put that down to my overactive imagination of always thinking the worse. It was December and the surgery was packed with both old and young with the majority showing signs of colds from hacking coughs to runny noses. I felt a sense of gratitude that I'd been blessed with robust health and had not been or felt ill for years. I then began to imagine my symptoms were a condition called mammary duct ectasia which would either disappear on its own or with a course of antibiotics, which I was not looking forward to taking. I had only taken antibiotics once before in my life so I guessed it would be gone in a week. Thinking beyond duct ectasia I also thought the condition may have been caused by having intimate relations with a man who had taken part in many clinical drug trials and this could be one of the side effects and my 'punishment'. Men who do clinical trials are advised to have protected sex for three months so this could be one of the undesired consequences.

The GP I saw and examined me suffered from Parkinson's disease so he found it quite difficult to evaluate his findings. His only words were "I hope it's not the Big C" and told me he would write and request an appointment at the local hospital for a mammogram. I was horrified, parts of the medical profession appear to have no real understanding of this illness, so little consolation or social decorum was offered at this time but looking back, the GP appeared quite fearful himself. The mind is a powerful thing, so plant the 'C' word into the mind of a potential victim and the seed is set to germinate, generating fear, stress and anxiety, bordering on complete panic. Add this to an already suppressed immune system and cancer may be ready to mutate into a tumour sooner rather than later. I managed to conduct myself with some dignity while leaving the surgery but then collapsed into a sobbing wreck within the confines of my car. Deep inside of me, I had obviously dreaded the worst and it was then my chaotic life finally came to a crashing halt. All other problems pale into insignificance when threatened with a potential death sentence like cancer. I remember driving home in a veil of tears ricocheting between self pity and incredible anger at God.

I took the following day off work to set myself up with the basics of a German anti-cancer diet I knew about. I could not afford to wallow too long in the powerless victim role so set about trying to take personal responsibility for the dilemma that I found myself in. All processed and refined sugar was to be eliminated because research has been seen to show that sugar actually encourages the growth of tumours. Meat, fish and diary were also off the menu as so many nutritional experts claim eating these 'carcinogenic' foods cause cancer. So a pretty Spartan diet had to be embraced. There was no time for self pity only action for healthy living and to continue as normal. Normal for me was healthy eating so it was of no great hardship but psychologically, I was at odds with this diet as a recovery tool. I knew many people whose diets were awful and they did not get diagnosed with cancer. My weight had stabilised for around a couple of decades maintaining a dress size 8/10. Exercise was a daily routine with healthy eating and cooking being a pleasurable pursuit. Drinking alcohol had never really featured big in my life because I do not like the feeling of being drunk and out of control. Losing days due to hangovers and alcohol induced illness is seen as a terrible waste of time for me. So had I been eating and drinking bad things that had finally manifested it into cancerous cells? No, a part of me knew the truth and the truth was simple, I was spiritually bankrupt. I'd been living a carcinogenic life in my head and heart so now the accumulated toxic thoughts must have finally manifested into this potentially positive cancer diagnosis.

The hospital appointment came a few days before Christmas however, on arrival at the clinic I was told that whoever conducts the screening was not around and that they would book me in after Christmas. I felt angry with this news after getting myself psyched up for this horrible appointment. Being kept in limbo until after Christmas was almost unbearable but I kept telling myself I would handle 'it' whatever the upshot was. My awareness and sensitivity had suddenly become much heightened since the C word had been introduced as I began to notice some obscure details at odd times. I noticed the breast clinic at the hospital is made to look like a spa with soft sofas, plants and coffee machines. I imagined the brief the interior designer was given when deciding on a scheme. 'This will be an area of the hospital where women will be given a possible devastating diagnosis so muted colours and soothing framed pictures may soften the blow.' Who were they kidding? I felt very cynical as I looked around, they may have thought this scheme may 'soften the blow' but I know nothing softens the blow of a positive diagnosis. Collapsing onto a wool carpet or a concrete floor makes no bloody difference. Those moments after a positive delivery diagnosis, is like free falling over the side of a cliff and I felt it wouldn't really matter if I hit the rocks or the sea.

Certain people in my life, once I'd told them cancer may be suspected, kept away from me under the guise they had a cold and did not want to infect me as that might compromise my immune system but I wasn't ill and never had been, I guessed they felt uncomfortable because they did not know what to say to me. Some did attempt with platitudes such as 'treatment has been making some advancements' but I did not want to hear it. Research had proved that treatment had basically stayed the same for the last few decades.

I went back to the hospital a second time in-between Christmas and New Year and had my first mammogram; I had always vowed I would never have one because I do not believe there is such a thing as safe radiation and more and more experts are claiming they do more harm than good. A book called Mammography Screening: Truth Lies and Controversy by Professor Peter Gotzsche explains this very clearly and is well worth a read. My experience of giving a child from Chernobyl a holiday in my home several years previously had taught me that I had just exposed myself to a massive dose of alleged 'safe radiation' by having a mammogram. But is there ever anything as 'safe radiation?' I don't believe there is, all radiation is damaging regardless of its diagnostic guise. An ultra sound scan followed, then without warning a local aesthetic was given for a biopsy. I didn't sign any consent for this form of invasive screening so the process somewhat immobilised me into silence. This is one of my major concerns about the diagnostic process; is that no one explains the procedures and the consequences of certain screening methods. I would have never consented or even allowed a biopsy knowing what I know now about 'seeding'. Seeding is the consequences of inserting a needle into the alleged tumour or lump. My understanding is that a tumour or lump is contained within a protective membrane however, once a needle is inserted this may allow the cancer cells to run rampant through the body creating a condition called metastasis.

Very similar to giving a dandelion clock a good blow. The doctor inserted the needle six times which was almost akin to grievous bodily harm. My GP who had Parkinson's disease had written to the hospital claiming he had found a lump the size of a hen's egg. This was due to his Parkinson's symptoms of very shaky hands. A more able GP would have categorically felt there were no lumps in my breast at all or at least nothing that could have been felt with a physical examination. I did not know this at the time but I guess the consultant was looking for this egg sized lump hence the multiple biopsies.

I asked the consultant what he thought I'd got, praying it was duct ectasia but he glibly answered my question with a question "what do you think you've got?" I could barely whisper the word "cancer" but he confirmed it with "you have cancer". I was horrified by his cold delivery and how quickly he left the room.

I dressed quickly struggling with the surgical dressings on my breast covering the puncture wounds, the nurse told me to take pain killers and that I would be bruised for several weeks. The doctors oath of First do no Harm came to mind but the thought disappeared as quickly as it came. I could feel the blood trickling down my midriff into the waist band of my trousers thinking how I would care for these wounds at home. Looking back now it's like everything was happening in slow motion, I remember crying quietly but questions screamed silently inside of me of how it had happened. Like many women I did not fit the typical breast cancer profile, positive health awareness had been my life. On my return home I just slumped into an unrecognised heap on the sofa while this information sank in. Curled up like a ball in the semi darkness refusing all food and drink, fearing I would just throw it all back up. Thoughts raced around my head like 'I don't want to die yet' and 'why me' to 'I must have done something really wrong to be punished like this'. The feelings of complete hopelessness almost consumed me. But I realised I had entertained thoughts of dying in the past when life's problems had got on top of me and I felt it was just these types of feelings that had now given me the cancer symptoms. So here I was again in a seemingly hopeless situation but doubly worse as the curse of cancer had been cast.

The next day I rang the help line the hospital gave me in case I had any questions. I asked how the consultant was able to diagnose before the pathologist's report had come back. The nurse explained that the consultant is an expert and he just 'knows' and if the biopsy results came back negative they would do it again until they find it. Like most authorities there's always an ego coupled with an air of 'we know better than you'. They may well do in that particular sphere of screening and alleged diagnosis but not in every treatment/recovery method. After talking with many women, I have now discovered that women can go back three to four times for biopsies until they find something. The nurse then continued to ask what exactly my concerns were, so I mentioned their particular type of treatment of surgery and possible radiation couldn't possibly be the only solution? She seemed astonished then she asked what my problems were with these forms of treatment; I replied with a long sigh "how long had she got for me to explain my concerns?"

I knew I'd be talking to a brick wall as I felt like an alien who had landed on a mad mechanical planet of robots who needed fixing with knives and chemicals. But I was a bloody human being not a robot and who was going to fix my broken psyche? Or jump-start my heart back into joyful living? The solution would not be found in the hands of a conventionally trained doctor or consultant. I had to keep reminding myself that I am not a machine but a unique individual so an identical treatment practice may promote recovery for some but others may simply die. I would not take the chance. Obviously the conversation ended there. Was I living in denial? I was hoping against hope 'they had got it all wrong' as so many hospitals do. They may have, as mammography is notoriously unreliable but I knew I'd never be told because the medical profession appear to have an almost 'god like' status where error or possible over diagnosis will never be admitted. But I knew I would never ever get on the allopathic cancer treatment conveyor belt of 'one size fits all'. After all I was not ill and was showing no signs of illness or experiencing any pain so I could live with this for a while until I could make an informed decision. I would not be bullied into accepting treatment that I know to be ineffective at least for me anyway. I sure had emotional pains but nothing physical but something inside of me told me if I accepted this treatment I would become very sick and would stay sick and weak for a very long time. This was not an option for what I still considered my healthy body. Maybe the NHS could put the money I saved them towards an OAP in pain who needed a hip replacement. I have since learnt that this is not the way the NHS works.

So I began to conduct my own research into various methods of treatment, initially they fell into two categories; downright barbaric or complete quackery.

I felt stuck between a rock and a hard place but I persevered because I refused to buy the current story of bodily destruction and death touted by the medical profession and the media. Several phone calls were made to alternative practitioners but most importantly to a lady I had met a few years earlier who had taken a non conventional route to treatment and recovery by going to Germany. She suggested we meet up and rationally discuss my next steps.

We met in a riverside café on a cold frosty morning; I must have looked like hell or an extra from the set of a Michael Jackson's Thriller video. She looked incredible, full of vitality, shining with health and so positive in her demeanour. A glimmer of hope began to appear for me as I considered going to the same place she had been. At this place in Germany I could strengthen myself physically and emotionally. Then I could face this diagnostic challenge that would enable me to make sound rational choices based on facts not assumptions or opinions. She also advised me to read a vitally important book written by possibly the most widely researched man on earth regarding cancer treatments. This man's name is Lothar Hernesie and the title of his book is 'Chemotherapy Heals Cancer and the World is Flat'

The book arrived by post on the morning of my official diagnosis back at the hospital. I took the book with me, not to spout sound bites from it because I was passed explaining myself to the medical fraternity. But I held it in front of my chest like a protective shield or talisman. Its information made me feel safe and supported. I had done some research and felt in a much better position to make an informed choice of treatment. As the consultant explained their findings, I began to feel disconnected from the room. My very kind ex husband came with me to observe the delivery of the diagnosis and ask any questions I might have forgotten to ask. But not much was asked from the hospital about me apart from name, address and bra size and did I smoke? But certainly no other lifestyle questions which has always surprised me. I have spoken with so many women diagnosed with cancer who had experienced some long term emotional and physical trauma several years before the onset of cancer. This leads me to believe stress and trauma may have a huge role to play in causing cells to mutate into cancer cells but nothing was asked about any of my 'contributing factors'. So if acute stress and trauma cause cancer, can living a peaceful but joyous life reverse the process? In the long term I believe it can. Then the ultimate doctors 'get out of jail card' question came, 'is there any one in your family who has suffered from cancer?' I confess to lying because I answered no, saying yes would have ended the conversation there and then with this easy genetic 'get out of jail' clause of no hope. I was on the brink of understanding epigenetics and the new biology so I did not want to buy the medical professionals story of being a powerless victim of hereditary. All my other questions on how I'd got it remained unanswered simply because the consultant did not know how to answer them.

The good news was that they had not found anything in the lymph glands but there was allegedly a small lesion behind the nipple. This could be removed by getting me in for surgery within three weeks, going on to reconstructive surgery and following up with radiotherapy if needed. I now understood why surgery is offered so quickly, they know biopsies disturb the cancerous cells and they need to act quickly by cutting away the offending cells. Radiotherapy is offered to be on the safe side (for them, not you). Chemotherapy or radiotherapy will always be offered to 'mop up' any stray cells created by biopsies and surgery as surgeons know cutting a tumour can encourage loose cancer cells to rampage around the body and possibly create a tumour somewhere else.

The usual cocktail of 'cut and burn' was offered before I had been given time to come to terms with what this diagnosis actually meant for me personally. It dawned on me that I was trying to seek a secure solution in a one track mechanical medical system and that may be the riskiest thing I could ever do in my entire life. I could not accept other people's opinions simply because they have a job title of GP, doctor, consultant, oncologist, specialist or whatever. I really needed to know the difference between treatment/recovery facts and treatment/recovery opinions. There does appear to be a very blurry line between facts and opinions especially in the cancer industry.

Some research shows that unless the tumour is big and is pressing on essential organs, surgery is not an option to be taken lightly. So while current cancer treatments may kill the cancerous cells it is incredibly detrimental to the rest of the body which could eventually result in death. I snapped back into reality and thought about all those people I had known that had died from treatment. It really did seem like I was being offered a huge sledge hammer to crack a nut.

The consultant was reading the back of the book I was holding which resulted in him looking rather ill at ease. I politely asked him for my notes because on this occasion I was refusing all treatment. The nurse behind him appeared agitated and asked what my plans were. I told them I would seek time and treatment in Germany. Research shows me that it takes several years for cancer to develop so a few months would not make a lot of difference. But I would be looking at this diagnosis from a different point of view and that is not to say one is better than the other. It simply makes sense to have more than one point of view when one's health and well being is at stake. The consultant was very gracious by stopping the nurse probing any more into my unorthodox plans. He shook my hand and wished me well for the future. Would he have really let me go that easily if the diagnosis was to be believed? Surely he had a duty of care to safeguard life? But no, I was out of there in several minutes with no hassle so maybe it wasn't that serious if I'd been released without warnings and admonishments.

Euphoric feelings swept over me as I waited for my medical notes to be collated for my imminent German trip. It was a Thursday, the sky was so blue and I suddenly felt free. Free of all the constraints of the medical world and totally independent to take responsibility for recovery and healing. I went back home, ate an unusually enormous hot vegetable casserole for my lunch and slept like a baby on the sofa.

On waking later that afternoon I took myself to the local travel agent and booked my flight to Stuttgart that was leaving in three days time. So after my initial knee jerk response of 'oh my God I'm dying sooner than expected' it then re-ignited itself into an automatic pilot of self preservation. That resulted in releasing me from all work commitments for the next 5/6 weeks. Some might say it was to 'lick my wounds' but I really needed to take stock and change my environment by retreating to the hills of Germany. A sense of guilt emerged in being diagnosed because I'd always been strong and robust in health and now I felt I'd let everyone down particularly my dad who had been worrying himself silly about me. But also I carried a strange sense of punishment that I deserved this diagnosis due to my 'unruly' behaviour and not sticking by my original marriage vows of being a good wife and mother. By changing the environment and distancing myself from painful situations did allow me the luxury to think about my next course of action for living life to the maximum.

That was to be the start of my journey into healing, recovery and maintenance treatments. It would be experienced both personally and on a deep academic level of scientific, spiritual and psychiatric understanding. History shows cancer to be as confusing as the definition of God. There are about as many authorities on cancer as there are on God and religion. Obviously each authority thinks their way is the only way. This proved to me that as an individual I needed to choose my diagnostic method and treatment plan very carefully indeed. This would move me beyond the constant fear to at least a partial acceptance that complete self healing is possible.

Chapter 2

MY ESCAPE TO GERMANY OUT OF HARMS WAY

Making the mind blowing decision to go to Germany was possible the scariest but also the most sensible thing to do at the time for my personal survival. I simply did not trust the medical system with my healing. It felt like a real escape as it was still dark when I took the very early morning train from Nottingham to London where I met my daughter. We travelled together to Heathrow on the tube train and I was so grateful for her easy company. I think we both sensed this was to be very exciting opportunity for healing and personal growth despite her own reservations. Saying good bye to her was terribly emotional for us both. She partly understood my decision to decline conventional treatment but as her paternal grandparents both used to work as medical professionals in the

NHS, her 'conventional medicine conditioning' ran deep. I had to keep reminding myself 'this cancer diagnosis is going to be a grain of sand, an irritant that will eventually create a pearl'. We both needed to hang onto that thought as we hugged each other at the departure gate in tears. I bet she never thought she'd be seeing her mother off to find cancer treatment in another country a few weeks previously. It's hard to even imagine the effect a cancer diagnosis has on a daughter but I think she knew deep down inside I'd handle it. I only hoped that she could handle it and trust that I would work out. But I physically hurt as she walked away to catch the tube back to London.

Boarding the Lufthansa jet almost felt traitorous, leaving the NHS behind to find recovery in Germany with unknown people suddenly appeared 'wrong'.

I arrived in Stuttgart in the evening and I felt very alone and scared. It was hard to grasp that I was in this strange unknown country because of a cancer diagnosis, something that I thought would never happen to me. But somehow this unique situation gave me a boost of hopeful energy because the thought of England and my old life only depleted me. Looking back life had appeared so mundane but also chaotic and lacking order from the scramble to earn money to a disingenuous relationship. I began to swing between elation and then despair remembering the drama and rejection. I felt like the past clung onto me like a bad smell permeating everything I did. My self respect was almost zero as I had tolerated stuff no healthy confident person would ever do. There had to be a better way to live. My first night in Germany was spent alone in a hotel near the airport before I could complete my last leg of the journey to my healing destination. It was dark and I felt very disorientated. The 3E Centre was situated in a mountainous region outside Stuttgart which was a few hours away. But it was in the hotel I hit bottom, I was hungry but so afraid of eating German 'carcinogenic' foods such as sausage and salami. I took a warm bath to quell the fear but the full force my desperate life so far had me trembling with terror as I lay in bed later trying to sleep.

Early next morning, still groggy with shock and disbelief that I was actually in Germany. I watched the neat German landscape flash by while on the train and I began to think that I was possibly beyond repair. I felt better seeing the morning dawn as I began to get my bearings.

Could this place really help clear up my psychological mess after a series of ongoing painful relationships and obsessions, which may have culminated itself in this rotten diagnosis? I felt pathetic and useless, a real sorry specimen of an ageing fifty two year old woman. The famous 12 Steps from AA had helped me clean up my life which I applied to an eating disorder I had 20 years previously. But cancer was different to an eating disorder, or was it? Maybe I'd never really recovered and simply swapped one insidious disease/condition for another?

Gazing from the train window, this part of Germany looked very different to the UK. It was clean, calm and orderly, possibly like England used to be forty years ago. As I watched the city give way to the countryside tiredness began to sweep over me as I realised I could not sustain this lack of food and nutrition any longer. I took a lone taxi from the station to the 3E centre where my confidence continued to diminish. Did I really believe this place could help me? My major disappointment was that Lothar, the author of the amazing book and owner of this place would not be here over the next 5 weeks and I would not get to meet him. I was gutted. To me he was the lynch pin of it all and I had been so looking forward to listening to his wisdom and passion. Glumness set in as I looked around at the other eight or so guests who were all female and appeared to be all German. I did not know a word of German and my loneliness increased. This was definitely the road less travelled and I knew I needed to change my mindset and quickly, for anything to work long term. After all these years spouting about holistic health, how could I ever choose the NHS allopathic route, surely I'd be a total hypocrite? I had to give this place a go, my life depended on it even though the place simply looked like a luxurious conference centre.

Some of the other guests/patients looked like they'd already had conventional treatment and it showed in their demeanour. I shuddered to think this could have been my fate if I had blindly and obediently gone down the conventional route. I had to believe my life is beginning anew and sincerely hoped wise guidance would be found here to make those changes I so desperately needed.

After a much needed nourishing lunch I settled into my very comfortable room and continued to read Lothar's book. It made me realise that it's all up to me, not 'them', not the doctors, not some miracle healer, simply me. Getting better or healthy was to be my responsibility, wow what a huge job. People and experts can show me the path but they can't do it for me. So the power has to be within me to get better. I'm finally coming to terms that I probably needed this cancer diagnosis for my previously undiscovered damaged psyche. My strong held beliefs told me that current conventional treatment would simply mask the symptoms and never get to the root causes. I had listened to others exalt their conventional doctors like they were gods but who the ***k were these so called humans after all? Some of these 'specialists' merely amputated breasts like a Red Indian who collects scalps. I thank God for my dad because without his financial help and ultimately his support I would not be here in this peaceful haven that began to resemble the perfect retreat for recovery.

The 3E centre is a large spacious modern building set in very tranquil rural surroundings close to the edge of an ancient forest. On the first full day we were given an individual plan of treatments and healing sessions but we were also given the freedom of choice whether or not to attend. We were told that they would not chase us around to force attendance. The days were still quite regimented with periods of walking and relaxation built into the schedule. After all, I was in Germany and it did have an almost military orderly professional edge to it. We were also advised never to chat about our 'illness' or previous treatments. It was deemed that this could have a negative effect on others which in turn could weaken the intention for healing...

Every day started almost the same way. We took part in the ancient eastern practice of 'oil pulling' which involves swishing organic sunflower oil around the mouth for 15 minutes then spitting it out. This harmless biological healing method improves dental health and apparently activates enzymes in the saliva which in turn draws toxins out of the blood. Many cases of breast cancer do have an oral hygiene link so this made a lot of sense to me. After a thorough rinsing we also drank a glass of sauerkraut juice which has to be tasted to be believed. This is an acquired taste but we were advised to persevere. This fermented juice contains a substance called isothiocyanates that may prevent the growth of cancerous cells. All of this was very new to me and I simply did as I was told, so what if sauerkraut juice tasted like fermented urine, it was still better than the conventional treatment back at home in the UK.

After a few days I began to wonder once again if the doctors in the UK had got it all wrong. Did I really have cancer? Maybe this 'illness' is not as easy to diagnose as the doctors would like us to believe. As we all carry cancer cells in our body, maybe it can only be arrested be never cured? Nothing is ever final except death of the body. So what if I subconsciously 'chosen' a cancer diagnosis as an opportunity to get mentally and spiritually well? No one here appears like a 'bad' person so surely cancer cannot be a punishment as I previously thought? Maybe it's simply a 'wake up' call to change my life path?

Later on that week we all had to see a conventional German doctor for a chat. I'm not sure why because much was lost in translation. After talking with the other women, it transpired that the doctor's wife had had breast cancer and had undergone a double mastectomy which I still call amputation. Anyway, I was told that he appeared to support the amputation of breasts suspected of cancer. I freaked out...f***king hell what a bombshell, I could have saved my money and time by staying in the UK. I really needed affirmation I was in the right place and doing the right thing because I was so bloody scared. Anger consumed me because this flew in the face of everything that Lothar had talked about in his book and the ethos of the place. As questions like 'after removing the breasts, does that mean cancer never returns?' Does it hell as like... I've known women whose cancer has come back with a vengeance even after both breasts have been amputated. I could not suppress my feelings for the sake of keeping the peace..."F**k you!" was running silently around my head as I sat across from this doctor. I categorically told him if this place and process is to prepare me for the inevitable surgery I may as well go home now. I was not happy; in fact I was furious and utterly deflated.

A decision had to be made as to whether I would spend the next month in this environment after the doctor's subjective opinions. I hoped that this medical maniac GP with his barbaric beliefs would not show his face again. Fortunately, he did not and allegedly his visit was down to German legal regulations that a registered GP had to be seen for the centre's licensing rules. As I mentioned much was lost in translation so I did not understand it fully but I feel that the centre could have made more of an effort to find a doctor who supported the aims of the place better. After my anger and fear dissipated I decided I would stay because 80% of what I saw suited my healing beliefs. The next person I saw was a doctor specialising in 'live' blood tests and it appeared mine was quite normal and healthy. I felt so much better compared to the previous days but I quickly realised nothing physical had changed only my perspective on my body. Positivity gradually crept in; I could finally see a future, a good calm future. Gratitude swept over me as I realised if I hadn't have gone to China four years previously on a business trip. I would have never met the photographer who took my photo for the local business newspaper, who originally told me about this healing place.

One of the only things that the 'mad' regulatory doctor had mentioned, that bordered on the esoteric, was that the cancer symptoms that showed in the left breast is the sign of a 'sorrowful' heart. Which was very interesting because I thought 'okay is it possible to turn that sorrow to joy?' Joy I'm still alive? Was I grasping at straws because I was still harbouring doubt and suspicion about this place? Who knows? The physical detoxing continued with the Budwig diet protocol, colonic irrigation, which I struggled with and daily coffee enemas. As I lay down to do my very first coffee enema, I felt revulsion but I had to keep reminding myself this has to be better than chemotherapy. That potentially damaging therapy has allegedly only a 2.2% contribution to the five year survival rate, 'stuff that' I said to myself; I knew chemo would never help me with my radical beliefs. At least the coffee enemas would not damage my heart, immune or respiratory system. At best the coffee would encourage my liver to dump toxic waste more efficiently and that in turn would unblock an important elimination point of the body. I had to go and read up in English to really understand the benefits. We were also encouraged to write and reflect on why we had been diagnosed with cancer as the condition is not random contrary to popular belief. But also to write how we were going to deal with good health.

My musings bought to the surface some of my greatest difficulties, one was the relationship starting with my mother. My earliest recollections were of fear and never really being able to do anything right. This led to a life time of alternating between calm 'people pleasing' that culminated into resentful inner explosive temper tantrums. Maybe my expectations of others had been too high because I felt constantly let down. I became needy and also desperate to be liked which made me hang onto relationships well past their sell by date. I believed at that time, anyone was better than being alone. It's only now that I realise this kind of self negating thinking and behaviour had the potential to kill me.

Money was also a massive contentious issue, I knew I had a poverty mindset even though looking back we were relatively rich as a family. Money and intimate relationships became intertwined as I dated very rich men or very poor men. The only middle ground I ever reached was with my ex husband who is the father of my only child. After that marriage failed I played the old familiar dating game again. Dating rich men ultimately left me feeling inferior and dating poor men made me feel pseudo superior. It was a strange recollection of thoughts now, looking back at the evidence in the cold light of day of my odd dating history.

After a week I began to feel more relaxed where periods of 'nothing to do, no where to go and no one to see' became the norm. Simply having quality sleep, good food, comfortable clothes and the institutional care began to feel like bliss. The five weeks seemed endless but I knew it takes 21 days to dismantle a habit so adding on an extra 14 days was for good measure in my eyes.

Tiredness began to catch up with me and I developed quite a headache which quickly became a migraine. This must be the result of the original trauma of being diagnosed to now being in the equivalent of the Garden of Eden all in the space of a few weeks. I was wiped out physically and mentally. I began to question why people who really abuse the physical body with alcohol and drugs don't seem to get cancer and it occurred that it may be a mental malady/sickness that manifests into rogue cells misbehaving, which is why I knew my solution would never be in medicine or hospitals.

Several things came up over the next few days that made me feel financially uneasy; one was the promotion of supplements in the form of intravenous vitamin C. The cost of them was around 170 Euros which made me feel uncomfortable and psychologically at odds. My symptoms were not a nutritional deficiency but an emotional malfunction. I had just begun to believe my body was becoming very powerful, powerful enough to generate health and vitality naturally. But I obviously still held onto a poverty mindset that I could not afford these injections. Secondly, my individual programme began to appear sparse and I also started to question the integrity of this place as at times I did not feel it was offering good value for money. But I did know my mind could jump from intense suspicion to a trusting naiveté which were both irrational and very annoying for me at times.

The mind work that was offered to me as an English speaking guest was a therapy called Time Line. This worked with the unconscious mind which included healing emotional traumas and eliminating unwanted thoughts, emotions and behaviours in minutes rather than days, months or years. My therapist was a delightful lady called Hannelore who had a real twinkle in her eye and the comforting demeanour of a favourite aunt. I always looked forward to seeing her as I became more and more willing to work with this process. She gave me access to tons of healing resources that I continue to use today as her suggestions were very wise. This part of the treatment became very important as I knew it was my mind that was defunct and not necessarily my body.

Being at the 3E Centre is in itself very therapeutic as the lovely energy around the building is so free flowing with high ceilings, lots of glass and natural timber surrounded by forest and countryside. The temperature always felt warm whilst the rooms were very cosy with snowy white duvets and big soft pillows. Anyone would surely feel better and rejuvenated spending time here. It always amazes me how people manage to get better in overcrowded hospitals. A place filled with contagious negative beliefs that focuses solely on sickness and drugs. Often denied of the normal and natural conditions of sun, fresh air, flora and fauna. Hospitals almost have a prison like existence. Throw in the processed reheated food, lack of privacy and medication and its little wonder that people do return over and over again. Possibly they almost never got truly well in the first place. At 3E we were almost forced to take back personal power regarding our own health and lifestyle choices. Obviously, this is a massive contrast to the conventional medical care where an individual is made to feel absolutely powerless who then have to put themselves at the mercy of doctors or nurses who in many cases; simply do not have the time or energy to promote real healing. If healing does occur in hospital, is that despite the system or because of it? I guess the answer lies in whatever belief system one might have and who is to be trusted with our health.

Anyway, I had to focus on my carcinogenic mind and heart and I certainly unearthed some toxic rubbish to do with forgiving others but also forgiving myself for the alleged mess I had made of my life so far. A day later this excavation of the mind gave way to a serious migraine that was so bad, the ambulance was called. Bloody hell, I could not afford to get tangled in the German medical system, after all I couldn't even communicate concerns to my own countryman who spoke my language let alone a foreign one. The paramedics checked my blood pressure and other things on site as I refused to get into the ambulance. I guess the emergency services had to be called as they could not be sure that the cancer had not metastasised to the brain. But I knew what it was, it was a migraine from total toxic brain overload and it was only afterwards I discovered if I'd done my coffee enema that morning it would have not occurred. Coffee enemas are touted as one of the most effective cures for migraine. It was after this incident that I discovered the care and affection from the other women being treated there, who were worried at my sudden withdrawal from activities and came to offer much needed support.

This chosen path of mine was not going to be as easy as originally expected but far safer than the conventional treatment back in the UK. Emotionally it was very painful and incredibly lonely at times. The not knowing and learning to trust myself again required great effort. I also experienced some vivid dreams where I could successfully make the link between dream memory and living memory. That in its self bought much release from the tight anxiety that had accompanied most of my life. Being at 3E after my shocking diagnosis now felt like falling in the proverbial pile of dung to be eventually coming up smelling of roses. My heart went out to all those people still receiving this diagnosis and not having the knowledge or resources to discover there are more healthier and natural choices. Yes, it takes courage to step out the system because once you 'know' it would then be very hard to opt back in.

The previous night we had been taught a spiritual folk dance by one of the other women there. As we danced by candlelight, I felt blessed by the intimacy of sisterhood but also by the fact that 70 years ago this healing experience would not have been possible in Germany. England was at war and these people were our 'enemies'. Thank goodness for Doctor Budwig who pioneered this treatment back in 1952 because there is still no place in the UK offering this type of holistic healing without trading standard officers crawling all over its back trying to implement the 1939 Cancer Act.

Part of me was half expecting a miraculous return to physical health with my breast returning to normal while I was there. But I knew I had much to learn and lots of negativity and odd beliefs to undo before this could happen and this would not happen overnight so I willed myself to simply live in the moment. That moment was healthy, peaceful and full of hope; I could be satisfied with that. That afternoon I attempted another colonic irrigation as I did not have a problem with these in the UK but here in Germany I found them very painful. The therapist was incredibly sensitive and kind but it felt like a real violation to my body. It reminded me of the suppositories that I had aged four after serious problems with constipation. I remembered that I could only defecate outside in the woods where I felt relaxed and never at home where I often felt tight with anxiety. I remembered then how dirty I was made to feel for doing this out in nature. Add this to wetting the bed for such a long time and being unable to speak at school because of a speech impediment it's no wonder I had felt such a failure. So the therapist stopped and gently massaged my feet for half an hour instead. On returning to my room, I sobbed for nearly two cathartic hours but I felt completely cleansed after the incident and released more negative feelings. I thought about my mum, she had died 16 years previously of cancer but I began to get glimpses of her and her sayings. One stuck in my mind "never get old" she used to sigh in one of her melancholy moments. Well she never did, she died at 54. I'm now choosing to spin that programming to keep myself young in spirit and not to follow the western inevitable path of degeneration once you pass a certain age.

I kept asking myself if I had accepted my current reality? The answer was yes and no, I still felt the doctors had got it wrong and that current diagnostic methods were notoriously unreliable. Was this denial? I remember the UK drug campaign a few years ago that said 'Just Say No'. I now felt that should be said about legalised drugs and pharmaceuticals that over exaggerate the beneficial claims and actually do harm like the sick making drug Tamoxifen. But I did 'believe' the original diagnosis had led me to take this powerful action towards recovery and change my life. So my current reality deep down at that time was still one of fear, anger, doubt and denial in spite of my sometimes fake Pollyanna attitude that everything is okay.

A gall bladder flush or liver flush was next on the agenda and this involved a two day fast. Much courage and tenacity is required to follow this one through to the end so inevitably only a few of us took part. I realised when the nutritional and social routine of taking food is avoided, time goes very slowly indeed. After the 48 hours had passed, a glass of half grapefruit juice and half olive oil has to be consumed before going to bed. Yuk, this was the real challenge. Also keeping the stuff down could be demanding. A medical member of staff stopped overnight in case of any dire consequences like puking it all back up. But typical to my usual form, I slept like a three logs as this mixture drizzled through my system. On rising, the following morning, I passed the equivalent of a half a kilo of peas. These were gall stones that had been softened by the consumption of apple juice and the delightful mix of grapefruit and olive oil. As queasy as this had made me feel originally, it still had to be better than surgery that some people have to remove gall stones.

All during the time spent here I had been having regular daily sessions from a Papimi device. This is a pulsed magnetic field generator that boosts the transmembrane potential of the cells by increasing the permeability to ions. This results in overall restoration and enhancement of the normal operation of the body. To me it felt like I had cleaned my 'energy' and reset my frequency to earth's frequency, which I believe to be at 7.8Hz. Normal healthy cells are around 70 millivolts; a tumour cell can be as low as 15 millivolts. This machine was energising the bodily electrical charge in order for the cell to become healthy again. At the time I took this machine for granted, it was only after a specialist came to give us a demonstration did I realise its incredible regenerating power.

Many of my personal beliefs were being called into question and I discovered most of them were not even mine. They had been inherited. So at the age of 52 it was time to choose my own that were more congruent with whom I really was. I had been told by my mum and some others, that if people really knew what I was really like, they'd be appalled... This perpetuated the sense of guilt and unworthiness. It was time to change that statement, so I wrote in my journal that if people really knew what I was like... wow, they would love me. Oh dear this felt fake and a bit extreme but I needed a jolt and not just the electrical one I got from the Papimi device.

The people I had chosen to surround myself mostly in the past also had low self esteem and that had aggravated me even more. So who did I think I was? Well, fairly talented and resourceful, a good person most of the time, a social asset, a loyal friend, passionate and a bit of a maverick. My new beliefs also included recovery is always possible, even more so for me because I am willing to do what it takes. Recovery and health is a state of mind not an end point and that health is always a personal choice. So I became determined not to allow others to hamper my healing with negativity and control. Healing is possible when a total adherence to personal truth is followed and I will succeed eventually.

However, a few weeks later, I felt that I had come to a spiritual standstill. I had 'believed' in God back in 1989 when I had a more childlike trusting approach which had been fostered by Christianity. But now my belief was simply riddled with insecurities and doubt, I just did not have a clue what to believe in any more. I had a concept of a 'life force' but did not know how to connect with a 'life force' that did not include pious petitioning and prayer. I knew my recovery was not simply contingent on nutrition or the regime; it was about my conscious contact with the 'life force' of my understanding.

So how does a clean living person like me get diagnosed with cancer? I questioned myself about all my clients who smoked, drank to excess, took legal and illegal drugs, only ate 'fast' greasy food and who sometimes had to be cajoled into taking a bath once a month or so. The whys whirled around my mind until I came up with my own subjective answer; what if all the above addictions and habits alleviated the stress so that there was no need to produce abnormal cells just to cope; BECAUSE they were already coping. Where I in my clean living world would never relax, never go on 'the lash' on a girls night-out simply because I'm too uptight to indulge in artificial sedatives and addictions. But maybe the artificial sedatives had 'saved' some people from manifesting the symptoms of cancer as we see more evidence is showing stress to be the main culprit of cancer. We all know and brag about someone who lived into their nineties and smoked 20 cigarettes a day without problems. But I had nothing to put in my empty anxious void, no addictions, not even organised religion so what could take the edge of my stress and anxiety?

Thinking about spirituality and religion again made me squirm inside. Some 'religious' people I had met and read about had at times displayed negative characteristics such as arrogance, self righteousness, pompous scripture spouting and patronising platitudes and so the list went on. I fell into the dark abyss of negativity but I felt I had to really feel these feelings so I could get beyond them. I had experienced feelings before like not being called a 'proper' catholic because I had been baptised into the Anglican Church. Also feeling judged when I shopped in certain areas or shops because I was not Moslem. I remember once going out with a Jewish man and many people telling me nothing would become of it because I was not Jewish. But it didn't just stop with religion as I used to feel guilty confessing that I did not watch the X Factor, Strictly or soaps, nor had no recognition of celebrities in magazines. I'm pleased to report this does not plague me any more as I do derive real pleasure from reading and scientific research instead. The courage was finally found to live an authentic life under my own rules and guidelines that are constantly being redefined. Being spiritual for me is what I do behind closed doors. Meditation has the amazing power to influence my life and perhaps the lives of others in ways I sometimes don't understand.

My mother had died when I was 35 years old. I had always thought my religion/spirituality/philosophy had alienated her. I used to believe it might have reunited us but when she died, my spiritual light definitely dimmed. I never really practised connecting with a 'life force' again. Life slowly went downhill culminating in a divorce and a destructive rebound relationship 10 years later. Looking back at the peak of my spiritual life, I appeared to have it all, maximum health, successful business, new marriage, beautiful baby and loads of friends. It did become increasingly difficult to be with my mother as the better I felt with my life, the sicker my mother became. I had believed that my wellness had possibly drained her health and ultimately sealed her death. Many people blamed me and still do for her demise.

The life coaching and therapy received at the 3E Centre really made me look at intimate relationships more deeply and examine my belief system. I had believed after my marriage had dissolved, meeting a good looking mature solvent man was nigh high impossible. The justification behind this belief was simple; many successful older men think they deserve someone younger and I had subconsciously set out to prove that point by dating men who always appeared to make references to young attractive women. So dating someone unsuccessful meant I would not be abandoned. This was crazy because I hardly looked like the back end of a bus, in fact far from it so obviously this belief in low self esteem had to be changed and changed quickly for a chance of a healthy future.

Money; now this was and still can be a contentious issue for me, sayings like 'money doesn't grow on trees' and 'you have to work really hard and be really clever to earn money' runs through me like the writing inside a stick of seaside rock. I felt anger at the 'rip off' society I currently live in; benefit fraud to self help gurus who charge exorbitant fees to attend workshops and seminars. I sometimes felt 'guilty' because I could have been seen to have more than others so I'd hide my success so no one could think bad of me. But I did come to realise this contentious issue could be turned around by looking at all the good things money and financial abundance can bring. At least I had the good grace to accept that I will never be a child protégée but it's never too late to be successful, whatever the subjective definition of successful is.

Getting back to the other guests at the 3E Centre, I came to the conclusion that some of the others appeared to be focusing on this protocol or that protocol. I felt disappointed that no one talked about the mental stuff, the stuff that put us in this place, the unresolved issues, and the emotional pain etc. No diet is ever going to fix that. Part of me was glad I did not speak German; it meant I could abstain from superfluous chit-chat that accompanied every mealtime. The day of silence we had certainly helped, freedom to simply be and discover inner peace. That was the day I became aware that the fear of dying left me, which meant I was no longer afraid to live. What a revelation, I could now embrace life in its entirety. I had always seen illness as a sign of weakness, almost pathetic. But survival is actually a sign of strength. Survival of the fittest does not mean an absence of illness but it can mean developing the strength to survive in spite of the illness. This cancer recovery has to be seen by our future generations as something that can be overcome. Recovery and healing has to be built into our children's psyche because if we succumb to death, we teach them we are powerless and that we have no control over degenerative diseases that are being peddled by the media daily. My message to my daughter is that one dimensional medicine can only help part of the way; the rest is up to you.

Being at the 3E Centre did not completely dissolve my fear as I was in uncharted territory and could not even contemplate the outcome. The day of silence produced some insights into the human condition. At lunchtime everyone wanted to sit in the same place which culminated in 5 people being squashed on one table while 3 people sat on another, why, because that is what they'd had always done and we weren't allowed to verbalise the justifications. The food which was amazing, still resulted in others toying and eyeballing it with suspicion because they were unable to get other people's verbal verdicts and talk through whether it was okay to eat or not. The sun was shining, good healthy nourishing food was being served yet many looked very miserable. I wanted to shout that they could always be in an NHS hospital eating micro waved shite masquerading as food? I actually saw someone who I knew was still drinking and smoking in her room spit out a minute piece of carrot and look at it as though it was poison. I laughed silently, the medical and pharmaceutical establishments need not worry about a mass exodus from the conventional system; 'they' know we're light years away from embracing this kind of recovery. Even some of the people here would perhaps better off in a conventional hospital.

I believe coming to the 3E Centre has saved me from a fate worse than death. I was not designed to run on one cylinder which is what the conventional treatment would have rendered me to, I was to be fully charged and firing on all four. I will accept the physical indication on my chest will continue to show until I have fully incorporated this new way of living into my whole life and that could take several years or not at all. I needed to protect myself from the political and medical scaremongering of diagnosing illnesses before they even occur. For me, cancer was a STOP sign in the the road. So how can certain treatments could be offered, if one does not know the cause? That still has me puzzled today? How did this even happen in this so called advanced intelligent world? Is like 'don't look at the cause, keep searching and waiting for the cure'. Society appears to have been dumb down from the contradictory medical propaganda in newspapers to the political/corporate narrative spouted on TV news shows by unelected non-experts.

If it seems as though I'm jumping from subject to subject, this is how my mind worked in this place. So much stuff was coming up that I felt compelled to just write as it came out. I was encouraged to visualize my new life back in the UK and write down my aims and aspirations. Again I am pleased to report most of them materialised within the year from getting a new car to a steady passive flow of income generated from some well researched investments in property. This came about by dropping the apprehension that had always plagued me, to opening my arms out wide to all the remarkable opportunities that came my way. I had always crept forward timidly when looking at new ideas knowing I could always shrink back and disappear. Not this time, I could boldly move forward with trust and accept the consequences, good or bad.

Some of the therapy offered at the 3E Centre could have been dismissed as quackery but this can be a ruse by medical professionals and their supporters to weaken the faith in healing naturally. There is a website called quack-watch, a very silly site designed to undermine and ridicule anything that does not fit into the big profit making pharmacy/medical world. I had to have the courage to stick with my convictions about this route I had chosen. Cancer was not diagnosed just because of food or environment or genes; it was through my toxic thoughts, plain and simple. My wonderful therapist, Hannelore really helped me 'wash' my mind of depressing thoughts. How would conventional medicine cope with that? Give me an anti-depressant pill or barbarically jump-start my mind with the still practised electric shock treatment?

I began to think about how medicine actually started. Doctors were the ones originally known as quacks selling all sorts of 'snakeskin oils' touted as cures. No wonder ancient healing women were labelled witches and burnt at the stake because these women knew the power of nature. They also had a passion and devotion to well-being without corporate profit driven agendas. The only passion I see in the huge 'sickness' industries is a desire for profit and keeping share/stake holders rich and happy. A few people are waking up and making enough noise to rattle a few cages within the pharmaceutical industry but a complete turnaround could take a very long time. Its easier to pop a pill than do this kind of work.

There are charlatans in many industries so the medical world is certainly not exempt. M. Scott Peck author of The People of Lie made a statement 'once a soldier had killed one Vietnamese woman and child, the next one became easier and the next easier still...' So it is with medicine, if they sometimes get it wrong, so what? Does it really matter to these 'not to be questioned' professionals if patients die from a misdiagnosis or wrong treatment? I guess not in the long run. If people really knew that they have the power to heal themselves there would be a recession in the pharmaceutical industry. But currently this industry calls the shots on politics, regulation and treatment funding. There are dramatic flaws in conventional medicine but they are definitely 'making hay while the sun shines' on people's continued ignorance and fear.

I had one more week left and was so looking forward to going home. It was not going to be that easy implementing my new knowledge at home but this was to be imperative for ongoing health. At least 10 books were read during my stay at 3E and the ones that held me close were the ones that encompassed quantum physics. They allowed me to see the mystery of being human in all its glory. Discovering and exploring the different systems of treatment had been very illuminating. I was now free to tailor make my own personal plan of recovery which was truly liberating.

As I returned my books to the 3E library I did want to remind the management to dump at least 70% of them, as they were about one dimensional physical treatments. Some appeared to glorify the sickness which completely missed the point that most illnesses are a mental malady. Many books took me 'around the houses' and never to the crux of the problem or the solution. Blind faith is okay in the beginning, now I wanted independent intelligence evidence that gives me autonomy and personal power. This would take time to integrate this into my new world but I felt excited about the future and its endless possibilities.

Going home back to the UK became a beacon of light. Seeing my daughter, my dad and my little dog (the three 'D's) became the focus of my attention towards the end of my stay. A close friend had booked a hair appointment and reserved a table at Nottingham's finest restaurant for my first proper night back. I was also looking forward to dressing up and being out socially for the first time in ages. So what did I see in this newly expanded world? Peace, serenity, financial flow, nurturing relationships, good health, continuing to look fresh and well and life's challenges being met with good energy and wisdom? A tall order maybe, but some of them would become a reality.

I was now on countdown and my thoughts had not quite stabilised. I tried to create thoughts of 'healing had already happened' but it felt like denial and denial is not recovery. I needed to accept my physical condition and work from there. A slightly retracted breast was not going to kill me but it did remind me on a daily basis that I had to accept this physical defect. My body was not my enemy; its physical manifestations were trying to help me by flagging up a mental malfunction. I was to accept my breast the way it was, without judgement which is a real challenge. No loathing, no disgust just respect for my body. My psyche has been through a long battle and my physical condition is an outward sign of all the damage that occurred. Acceptance has to be the key to recovery because without acceptance nothing can ever be changed.

The results of another 'live' blood test were given and things looked quite good. I wanted more but what did I expect after only 5 weeks? Working through an eating disorder over 20 years ago took about 9 months to be physically straight but at least 2 years to be mentally straight. I had an awful lot to be grateful for after all, I am still whole, healthy, energetic and fairly youthful looking. I knew I could continue with this nutrition programme indefinitely as it was of no great hardship. Many tools had been acquired to combat my resistance to healing. Fighting cancer was no longer an option as it kept me focused on cancer and like always attracts like, there are no exceptions. My focus is on healing, recovery and going with the flow. Reading a good book, cuddling my little dog, walking in the sunshine are all good soft fuzzy things that encourage healing.

The day of departure finally arrived and my work was done here. I felt nervous about returning to the UK and people asking questions about this form of treatment. We were given a pep talk about self protection which was basically not to waste time and energy with people who were sceptical or derogatory. We were reminded we did not need to explain ourselves to anyone. Fond goodbyes were said and addresses exchanged as I bundled my luggage into the waiting taxi. I realised this was the first time in 5 weeks I'd been out properly in public. The taxi dropped me at the station where I caught the train to Stuttgart airport. The flight was easy and uneventful but on arrival at Heathrow I noticed a dramatic change in the atmosphere and it was not related to the cold dampness of the British weather.

The place was so chaotic and full of people, the tubes had stopped working on the Piccadilly line for a while and the tension was almost palpable. As I crushed into a tiny standing space between construction workers and my luggage, I could hardly breathe, I thought 'welcome home, welcome back to the chaos. My daughter was waiting for me at St. Pancras and it seemed like no time had passed since we last met as we hugged each other. It's easy to forget the effect this has on loved ones because they are also susceptible to the fear-mongering of aggressive medical marketing suggesting death and bodily destruction is inevitable. She remarked on my good health and that it looked like I'd just returned from a spa. But looking and feeling like this is what health and healing is about. Returning with a body that resembled the terrain of The Somme was NOT recovery. I think when she saw me she felt relieved I was simply alive and in one piece as I had been unable to describe this healing treatment over the phone. We had a drink together as I attempted to tell her about my stay but I had no words that could sum it up at that time. We hugged again before I caught the last train to Nottingham. My dad was waiting for me on a cold snowy platform, he embraced me back into my life with relief written all over his cold face. It's alright doing this healing protocol in an organised treatment centre but could I really continue this back into everyday living and achieve permanent recovery?

Chapter 3

LET FOOD BE THY MEDICINE

There are so many approaches to nutrition where illness is concerned but finding the right individual plan and staying with it takes a lot of courage and tenacity. I'm still not sure whether my chosen food plan was courage or sheer bloody mindedness. But I believed it would give me a better chance than anything else I'd looked at and it certainly would not harm me. Doctors and nutritionists appear to be at opposite ends of the spectrum where healing foods are concerned but not only that, each and every nutritionist offers a different theory thus confusing us more than ever. If personal doubt is ever entertained as to whether or not the right diet or protocol is being followed just listen to a few nutritionists/experts and one can soon be thrown off track as I was many times. The secret is finding a plan that feels comfortable coupled with enough scientific evidence to alleviate doubt that will ultimately offer the best chance for a strong recovery start. A cancer diagnosis can create so much fear which is why it's relatively easy to question every personal decision made regarding treatment plans and because I did not initially have enough information it appeared like I was questioning everything. This can get tricky if others keep asking exactly how it works and you're not really sure how to explain the science behind it or give them cold hard convincing evidence.

Coming back to the UK was like coming back to a different planet after my pure healing energising foods I had consumed in Germany. Sticking to the Budwig protocol became the primary focus of my life as it seemed that was all I'd got left to hang onto. I had not yet grasped the full meaning of recovery so the diet became my life raft. Ordinary food scared me, there appeared to be so much sugar, so much fat, so many carcinogens, how would I ever survive now I did not eat like 'normal' people? Simply staying on this protocol and screening out other theories did eventually become so empowering because I was actually doing something and taking responsibility for my own body. It seemed the least I could do whatever happened. In the beginning I was met with a lot of scepticism and sometimes badly disguised ridicule as I refused all food that did not fall into my Budwig category of allowed foods.

The main staple of the Budwig diet is the flax seed oil or linseed oil (as some call it) and quark mixed together. This base mix has ingredients added to it to either make it sweet or savoury.

Fortunately, I found this part easy as the mix is so delicious. Breakfast is certainly no hardship as freshly ground flaxseed, cinnamon, honey and fresh pineapple is stirred into the first mix of the day. I have been admonished by several nutritionists for eating diary, especially after being diagnosed with breast cancer but I tell them the mix forms a lipoprotein so it's no longer a singular diary item. I ask them to research the science but no one ever does that because it's easier to believe in what they've always believed in. But from my understanding the quark becomes a carrier as it binds with the flax seed oil. Flax seed oil contains masses of oxygen but the oil is unable to penetrate the cancer cells directly. Quark enables the oil to emulsify and only then can the oxygen rich properties get into the cancer cell. Cancer cells apparently hate oxygen and for this reason the Budwig diet appeared to be the only sensible diet to follow based on my biological beliefs. This biochemical food mix contains both proteins and lipids. This somehow this allows the fats to move through the water inside and outside the cells including the cancerous cells. Whatever the science, I knew it increased my energy and vitality but my inquiring mind wanted to know why and how because this could simply be a placebo.

Back at home on my own computer I set about learning as much as I could about Dr Johanna Budwig. The results astounded me; this wasn't some vague esoteric housewife floating about mixing foodstuffs together in her kitchen to create a magic potion. Dr Budwig was born in 1908 and died in 2003 aged 94 and was possibly the world's leading authority on fats and oils relating to cancer. Unfortunately, there is no official successor. She was the

German Government's senior expert on fats and pharmaceutical drugs, she was a cancer research scientist, a blood specialist, a pharmacologist and physicist, and to me she was an angel. Tears of gratitude can still well up inside whenever I look at her photograph because she was the beginning of my healing; restoring hope from my initial despair. In spite of her medical background she believed the usual conventional treatments for cancer can lead to a worsening of the disease or a speedier death and in healthy people, can quickly cause cancer. This was music to my ears as so many people looked at me askance whenever it was mentioned that I had refused conventional treatment and was taking responsibility for my own recovery.

What my original non-science mind managed to pull from this protocol was that certain fats were indeed detrimental to health and even more so if attempting to recover from a degenerative disease like cancer. It had dawned on me a few decades earlier that what most people put in their supermarket trolleys was in fact processed product and not real food produce. Packaged, canned and frozen food had always appeared as dead food to me. Back in the early 90's I did become an avid campaigner against hydrogenated fats that seemed to be in most food products. I saw no nutritional value in this substance as it appeared to be inert and allegedly taxes the liver when trying to break it down in the digestion process. Only then I had little knowledge of the science and why it caused so many malfunctions in the body. Its only asset appeared to be is that it prolonged the shelf life of food stuffs thereby increasing profits for the food manufacturers. What I've since gathered is that there's a lot more to fats and oils than I ever imagined. There's a book called 'Fats that kill, Fats that heal', I really recommend reading this book to discover the reasoning behind why we've been fed fraudulent information about the consumption of margarine and shortening. It will explain in detail why a fine balance of oils that include essential fatty acids is critical to good health and a long life.

When I asked the doctor who delivered my diagnosis if there is an anti-cancer diet, he said no and it seems most doctors will invariably say no and basically tell you to carry on as normal. But what is a normal western diet, lots of highly processed fatty foods and sugar? Both these things are dangerous to health but even more so if one is diagnosed with cancer. Why do so many doctors fight against anti-cancer diets? One possible reason could be because nutrition is not studied when training to become a doctor? Or perhaps they know that diet is only a small part of the solution and seeing a psychiatrist as well could offer more hope? So maybe some ideas are always rejected when one doesn't quite understand the subject. Or it could be the 1939 Cancer Act which in a nutshell, stops doctors talking about any other treatments outside of conventional treatments. There are many other conclusions that I have come to but I am choosing to believe that you always oppose some ideas that you don't fully understand or have not studied in depth. There may be more sinister agendas such as 'cancer is a very profitable industry' and finding out that cheap natural alternatives may heal cancer is something that has to be kept quiet. But these types of thoughts do not help my personal healing as I need to focus on the positive and what really works on a practical level for the health of my body and mind.

When I continued to press the doctor who diagnosed me, if there was anything I could do to help myself, he flatly declared there was nothing anyone could do and almost snorted with derision that nutrition could have any answers. A saying that sprung immediately to my mind was 'save your contempt prior to a thorough investigation' after that particular dismissive response was thrown in my direction. I genuinely thought the doctor could advise me on what I could contribute myself to keeping the diagnosed symptoms at bay or even what I could do to strengthen my immune system but nothing was forthcoming. It was like the doctor was claiming only he had the power to 'help' me. But help me towards what? Healing and recovery? I think not. It was at that moment with utter confidence that I was able to walk away from the national health care system. But I have to admit that sediments of disappointment remained with me over the doctor's ignorance and lack of knowledge about the proven alternatives that offer a more gentle approach to recovery.

What is most startling about all of this is that the doctor's role appears to be a very disempowering process for the patient. It places all the emphasis on their standard procedures into bullying the body for a response. Notice I say a response rather than healing because standard treatment does indeed prompt a response but certainly not the one I would like to experience. This provoked me into studying what a potential doctor is actually learning at medical school. Even the word medical has everything to do with medicine and sickness. It's a pity there is not a 'health' school that focuses on how healthy people stay healthy or what prompts some people to live and some to die even though they can submit themselves to the same treatment. I guess there would not be much profit in that as natural remedies cannot be patented. Disease is a better business model and the 1939 cancer act ensures that no one else is allowed to compete outside the medical system. We need a free market where medicine is concerned that could be cut loose from corporate monopolies. Its an unequal playing field with many injustices. And they still call this democracy. Tony Benn a British politician once said an educated, healthy and confident nation is much harder to govern than a hopeless and pessimistic one and perhaps I should add a sick nation. So maybe there is an agenda behind it? So many patients may die from standard treatment and not from the actual cancer itself. A doctor appears to have had little or no training at all on nutrition. The education is 'disease oriented' with an incredibly heavy emphasis on the use of pharmaceuticals. This is where a doctor learns about drugs and why and when to use them with the usual backward approach of fighting the symptoms whilst remaining ignorant to the cause. Doctors get paid for treating, not for curing diseases. But at the risk of repeating myself over and over again, 'a body can never be drugged or bullied back into health'.

Cancer was virtually unknown 100 years ago possibly because people used food in its original form, always in season and as close to nature as possible, thereby maximising healing. But there are some really weird products out there now masquerading as food and it appears hardly anyone is exempt from the consequences of this highly processed food industry. I had always tried to consume a healthy diet maintaining a normal weight for my height and frame over the past couple of decades. My skin and hair always looked fairly healthy and youthful despite my pinched anxious expression that had occupied my demeanour some of the time prior to diagnosis. So imagine my horror seeing my own live blood test for the first time; my red blood cells were all stuck together like a stack of chocolate buttons. Apparently this is not healthy; the cells should be singular and free flowing which allows for the body and blood to always be oxygenated. Red blood cells clumped together is a sure sign of some malfunction in the body, so the inevitable result of oxygen depleted cells coupled with ongoing stress has to be a positive cancer diagnosis. How many people would show these precursors to cancer if tested? My guess is many but this is relatively simple to reverse with the correct diet and lifestyle. The diet and lifestyle I had was still relatively healthy compared to the modern western diet consumed by many people today but I had still shown these oxygen depleted 'sick' cells despite of it.

Doctors in the UK still publicly refuse to accept sugar could be related to cancer but after my initial informal diagnosis I decided to eradicate all white sugars from my diet as much as I could. A tumour's fuel of choice is glucose so it makes sense to stop consuming white sugar if faced with an alleged life threatening disease. I have since discovered that doctors and scientists are aware of tumours attraction to sugar because there is a new chemo drug that is hidden within a 'sugar Trojan horse'. This will deliver a shot of chemo directly to its target, namely the tumour which gobbles up the sugar but also the chemotherapy agent hidden inside. Sugar is addictive but it is addiction by stealth as it appears in many processed foods and not just sweet foods but as many savoury foods now contain sugar. Many supermarket aisles could be renamed as confectionery. I remember picking up a salad in a high quality supermarket chain and one of the main ingredients was sugar. It saddens me that sugar has to be added to make salad and greens to make it more appetizing. Tumours 'high-jack' glucose/sugar and block oxygen, so the tumours can get bigger but no one talks about this tumour growing substance called sugar especially in the medical profession. Again sugar is another massive industry and sugar's cheaper alternative, corn syrup that is found in many 'fast' foods and drinks is as equally addictive and destructive but also incredibly profitable. Surely if someone diagnosed with cancer were told 'actually sugar may make the cancer worse', would you still consume sugary foods? My guess is possibly because sugar is as addictive as nicotine and some cancer medications and treatments can actually create a yearning for instant energy foods which is where sugar products step in. One person I knew diagnosed with breast cancer that used to be slim, began to consume huge amounts of sugar as in boiled sweets once on steroids. She ballooned in size and eventually died at 38 years old. As only one major cause is allowed on the death certificate it had to go down as cancer but the treatment and the subsequent consequences of treatment, I believe caused her death.

I then began to get interested in the little things that really contribute to real health, for instance the correct intake of magnesium, calcium, sodium and potassium. With this knowledge I was able to understand why my daughter had had a predisposition to childhood eczema and asthma after her childhood vaccinations. I know now that I did not drink enough water whilst pregnant and was possibly chronically dehydrated. It was with interest that I learnt that an imbalance of these electrolytes may cause the placenta to be in the wrong position resulting in all kinds of birthing problems. I never realised how important nutrition really is when trying to create a new healthy life.

It was with great sadness that I watched the documentary of Kaiser Wilhelm II. He was born presenting breach which indicates his mother, the Empress Victoria was lacking in vital nutrients. Adequate nutrients ensure the placenta moves upwards allowing the baby more room to turn. Unfortunately, the attending doctor pulled Kaiser Wilhelm out by his arm. Consequently, he then suffered a permanently paralysed arm. In 1859 and being royal this was seen as shameful and he was rejected by his mother. He went on to endure years of horrific treatments. None of this was his fault but he was made to feel inferior, less than perfect which led to his very dysfunctional erratic behaviour. This may have led to the obsession with his mother which she chose to ignore. So after his father died of throat cancer he chose to blame the English doctor while still remembering it was an English doctor that had crippled his arm. His hatred of the English may have led to the triggering of

WW1. Imagine if he had been born perfect and his mother had loved him, would WW1 have reached the devastating conclusion it did? This I will never know but if a doctor ever claims nutrition has no effect, just look at what might have happened if Queen Victoria's daughter's nutritional needs had been met through a wise sage specialising in natural health, instead of seeing something as natural as giving birth a medical condition.

A friend told me her two year old grandchild had been diagnosed with cancer. It turned out the child's diet had been particularly bad but had actually got worse after diagnosis and treatment. The child had not really eaten any real fruit or vegetables in its entire short life. After discovering cancer and the ensuing treatment, the focus was on quantity and calories so with medical guidance, the parents allowed the child to eat McDonald's doughnuts (sugar) and sausage rolls (densely heated fats). So whilst these foods are fun once in a while they do not constitute nutrition for a sick child diagnosed with cancer. My friend went onto to say that the muscle wastage had to be seen to be believed as no one had emphasised the importance of protein for a growing child. The child had sat slumped on a sofa watching cartoons on the TV all day in some kind of hypnotic state probably going through sugar highs and lows. The child is still unable to walk. Is this child abuse? I guess it is but will never be seen that way by any government authority in this country. My hope is that the child's spirit and will to live is strong enough because there appears to be little else helping towards healing and recovery.

My understanding increased as I realised that the oil protein diet that Dr Budwig advocates is more than nutrition; it takes into consideration electromagnetic stresses (smart meters and mobile phone towers) caused by modern day living and other mental stresses we can all subject ourselves to. Budwig is known to have said 'she could help a woman recover from breast cancer but if she returns to a wife beating husband there is little hope for recovery'. This made me realise how important my mental health is in regard to long term recovery. So whilst medical experts claim there is no anti-cancer diet it does makes common sense that anyone with positive mental stability would not abuse their precious bodies with junk food. But who has a positive frame of mind whilst coming to terms with the initial diagnosis of cancer? This is why I knew it is even more important for the body to adopt a healthy eating plan immediately if one is attempting to heal from a degenerate disease like cancer. Even if the reason for following the diet, was to take focus off sickness for a while and turn to health. A healthy body also responds more positively to conventional cancer treatments too.

We are heliotropes apparently (beings who respond to the stimulus of sunlight) and just like plants that naturally turn to the light we need to get the best from natural daylight. Sunlight and unsaturated fats complement each other but the less light there is, the more we need essential fatty acids. Eating too much margarine, animal fats and highly heated oils found in many processed convenience foods steal precious electrons from the body. Radiation and chemotherapy are also known as electron stealer's. The presence of essential fatty acids in our body ensures that photons of sunlight are absorbed as energy. This is for future use in important biochemical reactions in our bodies and the vitamin that can restore this process is vitamin D3.

Vitamin D is sometimes called the sunshine vitamin. Whilst in Germany we were told to go outside twice a day for a walk and a dose of vitamin D. It was winter so wrapping up warm and sitting on a bench for at least 20 minutes was incredibly beneficial. My favourite comedian Peter Kay jokes about his dad, when finding his kids inside watching television with the curtains drawn on a sunny day, would shout 'get outside, it's sunny, don't waste it'. Peter Kay's dad probably did not know that humans are heliotropes and that vitamin D from sunlight activates the immune/support system, he knew it intuitively. Without vitamin D the immune system's fighter T cells remain dormant. But Peter Kay's dad did inherently know that sunshine is indeed very beneficial and possibly did not want a bunch of sick kids lying around in the summer holidays unable to go back to school in the September through lack of sunlight.

We may laugh at many of the things the old folk say but inside these funny sayings lay ancient wisdom which is passed through the generations. I do love Peter Kay and he is one of my many healing tools, I'm not sure how he'd take that statement but I'm sure he'd make a wonderful joke from it. But he makes me cry with laughter which I know releases good feeling chemicals from my brain which in turn strengthens my immune system. Some people have been known to laugh themselves back to health.

Getting back to vitamin D, I since discovered people suffering from cancer almost always show a vitamin D deficiency. A study published in March 2010 issue of the Journal of Clinical Endocrinology and Metabolism found that a staggering 59% of the population is vitamin D deficient. So now that evidence has shown vitamin D activates the immune system, how can any vaccine work without a strong immune system to respond to it? Not only that, we are being constantly scared off staying in the sunlight by skin cancer advertising campaigns over exaggerating the perils of sun bathing. Whilst over exposure is very dangerous, constant lack of sunlight may be another 'trigger cause' behind so many degenerative diseases. Many people in today's modern society live, work and play indoors, nearly always under artificial light and this can cause severe deficiencies. A friend who has undergone several rounds of chemotherapy is always advised to keep out of the sunlight. Chemotherapy and radiation can make the skin sensitive for several years and much advice is given by cancer organisations to basically never submit skin, head and eyes to natural sunlight again. This to me, questions the boundaries of sanity. Sunlight can help prevent approximately 77% of ALL cancers so by avoiding chemical carcinogens, high levels of trans-fats and increase the dietary intake of plant-derived nutrients, the body can indeed help itself towards healing. As I live in the UK, sunlight can seem like a rare occurrence so I do supplement my diet with vitamin D3 sometimes taking up to 10,000IU's on short dark winter days. Anyone who suggested that I avoid sunlight because they had put poison in the form of chemo in my body that now made me allergic to sun; I would consider them being very ignorant to the basics of life. Please excuse my anger as it seems these barbaric treatments are designed to destroy even the simple pleasures of life. Being on a beach with the warm sunlight and fresh air caressing limbs normally encased in garments has to be bliss for me. Take a plant indoors and preferably put it in a cellar, feed it with chemicals and watch it eventually shrivel and die. Cancer treatment victims can sometimes look like shrivelled plants, call it vain but I'd rather stick with a short but a quality way of life with sunshine and the ability to enjoy good natural food than die in this hopeless undignified way. I believe this is covert violence which I see as a medical crime. So in the conventional cancer industry sunlight is bad and chemotherapy chemicals are good, food is useless and pharmaceuticals are essential. A cancer diagnosis is not due to a lack of chemotherapy or other drugs. Wow, how did society get brainwashed into some of these ridiculous inverted ideas?

In Germany I had received the best quality organic ingredients but now I was back home these basic staples were proving difficult to find. I used to order the staples direct from Germany but the doctor no longer offers this service. There are some pretty good fresh oils and alternatives in UK production. But being back in the UK, I soon discovered the food was the least of my problems. 'Be fearful of cancer' advertising was everywhere, jingles appeared on the radio promoting the latest symptom to look for and always urging you to go for 'free' screening as soon as possible. I had learnt so much in Germany but the fear always reared its head when I saw these propaganda adverts. The fear became interchangeable, first it was food and the diet then it switched back to cancer and who did I think I was kidding by refusing the poisonous treatment offered by conventional medicine? My fear began to show itself in the anxiety about eating out or going to someone's home for dinner. I did feel neurotic and stupid constantly asking for a rundown of the minute details of ingredients in every morsel of food. I knew I had to change my thought process or the stress around food and eating could cause more problems than it would solve.

My life at times began to shrink; I did not want to be focusing on the bloody cancer diagnosis all the time. By continuing my research I soon discovered foods by themselves, are not carcinogenic contrary to what the nutritional experts would have you believe. What I have since come to believe that if care has not been taken with nutrition leading up to the diagnosis of cancer then these so called 'bad' foods may 'piggyback' the already present condition of cancer. This did not stop me trying and testing nearly everything that claimed to cure cancer. I had already read about the amazing properties of turmeric and so it did not come as a surprise when I heard on the local TV news station that some researchers at the Nottingham Queens Medical School were conducting some trials on the benefits of turmeric and chemo. My first thought was dump the chemotherapy; the turmeric will work all by itself. But turmeric does reduce some of the negative effects of chemotherapy. Turmeric is a natural anti-inflammatory but from a western medical point of view the evidence is not strong enough yet, so I'm hoping this research throws up some real medical evidence soon.

I have become quite well known at my local Asian supermarket where my search for fresh turmeric finally ended. This amazing root spice actually increases its potency when mixed with freshly ground black pepper corns. I couldn't believe that fresh turmeric is so incredibly cheap. I originally did not know what fresh turmeric looked liked until I snapped open a 'twig like' looking spice and revealed its amazing orange coloured interior. Powdered turmeric is just as good as I often use this as part of a simple but very tasty salad dressing. Many studies have been conducted that show turmeric can induce a process that triggers the self destruction of cancerous and damaged cells. The main component of turmeric is curcumin which is very powerful and is one of the best things you can add to a diet for long term health.

Many people asked me how long I would have to stay on this diet and I would answer "for as long as I wanted to live well", this would be seen as rather provocative for some but I do love this diet. Its healthy, it's natural and delicious and it suits me. I now understand the science behind it which strengthens my body's intention for healing.

Fear can be quite insidious because even with all this knowledge on food and diet, thoughts kept jumping back to 'what if I'd got it all wrong'. It was then I realised it was nothing to do with the food but my mental state of mind. I had started to write this book and the courage to finish it was diminishing fast as I believed I had no real conclusion or resolution. Family members kept asking when I was going to go for another thermal scan,

I said I did not need one yet as screening would have increased my anxiety levels even more. Going for a scan, any kind of scan/test in a state of fear is not a good idea as it increases adrenalin and cortisol. I wanted to go with an attitude of peace and a strong belief that I was doing okay so that my body resonated with health.

It was at this low point I came across an amazing book written by a Chinese psychiatrist and doctor called Tien-Sheng Hsu. This book ironed out all the wrinkles in my developing awareness about healing. What I read, I knew but had never seen it written in this way. I would recommend reading The Secret to Healing Cancer; it puts the disease of cancer in perfect context and helps anyone reclaim their power. My level of consciousness is now quite high, I appear to intuitively know what foods can be handled by my body and what foods can't. It all depends on my mental state, for instance I would not choose to comfort eat during stressful or upsetting times. This would be very detrimental to my physical well-being and would be seen by my body as a punishment. I choose to increase my water intake in times of stress. I still choose not to eat too much white sugar and will occasionally have chips. When eating out, I'm usually with friends so I generally have a happy attitude. This allows my body to process the portion of fish and chips with a positive attitude without guilt so it has no negative effect on my body. This natural protocol of eating has definitely jumped started my healing process and nature does provide an amazing array of healing foods so it has to be a good place to start.

Eating respectfully for my body is all about responsibility and that is only something I can do. I knew my conventional diagnosis did not represent the big picture and was purely an assessment of a tiny part of my body that had decided to flag up a psychological malfunction and manifest as a physical lesion. I also knew that almost every cell in my body renews themselves every few weeks so surely with the right nutrition and the right frame of mind I could correct this lesion? Well I was certainly prepared to try it even if it took years, what could I possibly lose? I wanted to live a satisfying life and this was only possible with a healthy body. A healthy diet became a firm foundation for recovery in a way that no medical or chemical intervention can ever do. I believe Mother Nature could be my healing guide to begin this empowering process.

INFRA RED SCREENING VERSUS MAMMOGRAMS

My next step was the attempt to measure the progress I had made and I believed the only way was through some sort of safe screening. By now and with the knowledge that I now possessed I knew I could not subject my body to ionising radiation found in mammography. Not only because of the damaging radiation but also mammograms are now being shown to be notoriously unreliable. Family and friends, possibly out of concern were pressing me to get some concrete evidence or a guarantee that would ensure I was on the right path. But life never really gives us any guarantees except death and taxes. But I set about researching all I could about alternative screening.

I do remember getting my first invite for a mammogram shortly after my 50th birthday. Even before I knew anything about cancer I had made a conscious decision to decline a mammogram and dumped the paperwork straight into the bin. My mother had had many mammograms and clearly stated how dehumanising it all was but she felt as though she had no other choice than to allow life negating radiation to crush the delicate breast tissue each and every time. I did not take much notice at the time as it seemed as though as I was light years away from all this medical screening malarkey. It was in 1991 however, a benign lump was discovered in my mother's breast and a 'just in case' lumpectomy was performed shortly after. She was allegedly given the all clear but it appeared she never really recovered from her ordeal. She was in pain with her lymph glands malfunctioning and she also developed an undiagnosed goitre. My mother died aged 54 from apparent lung cancer (she never smoked) 24 hours after being diagnosed.

Was it cancer that killed her or the shock of being diagnosed or the disfiguring surgery? My mum had had a history of ill health and had battled with each and every ailment so could she have decided to simply give up? Fighting an illness is very draining and time consuming. She may have also believed that's all there was left, the long fight back with all its inevitable medical interventions. Unfortunately our archaic system of diagnosing illness is always focused on aggressively fighting illness once it's discovered. I knew I never wanted to 'fight' for my life as that would always bring me more of what I didn't want. Morbidly looking for sickness in whatever guise it comes in, will always in

my opinion, eventually bring sickness. I wanted health, robust
health and so wanted to stay focused on health and only health.

On my initial discovery that something may be wrong with
my breast, it still took me three months to seek advice. So
it was with great trepidation that I actually made that first
appointment to see my GP. After the GP looked at my slightly
retracted breast he obviously advised going to the hospital for
my first mammogram. I really didn't want to do this but I went
anyway. The mammography room at the hospital was in semi
darkness, which appeared a bit spooky and I remember looking
with horror at the huge electrical unit on the wall. This unit
was responsible for emitting huge doses of ionising radiation
to mainly innocent delicate female breasts including mine. As
I removed the clothes from my upper body I couldn't believe
I was actually subjecting myself to this hideous ordeal that
could possibly be causing cancer if I hadn't already got it. A
mammogram is an actual X-ray so I knew I was now exposing
myself to dangerous radiation that is probably ten fold more
powerful than a normal chest X-ray. It's strange that Ms Patnick,
co-ordinator of the NHS Breast Screening Programme claims
"sixty percent of screening detected cancers are in women
returning to us for repeat screening". Duh, isn't this giving us an
indicator that repeat screening may indeed cause cancer? I'm not
too sure I would shout about that as Professor Peter Gotzsche,
leader of the Nordic Cochrane Centre has been analysing the
real benefits of mammograms for a decade and his findings are
pretty scary. He claims through 'science based evidence' that
the most effective way to decrease a women's risk of becoming

a breast cancer patient is to avoid screening. He goes on to say mammography screening is one of the greatest controversies in healthcare, and the extent to which some scientists have sacrificed sound scientific principles in order to arrive at a politically acceptable result in their research is extraordinary. In contrast, neutral observers increasingly find the benefit of mammography has been much oversold and the harms are much greater than previously believed". Routine mammography for example (two x-rays on each breast) is the equivalent to having a 1000 normal chest or spinal x-rays. Even Professor Michael Baum who helped set up the NHS screening programme claims that mammograms are doing more harm than good. The debate continues on and I would advise anyone contemplating a mammogram to keep them selves up to date with current unbiased research before subjecting themselves to this particular potentially 'cancer causing' diagnostic tool. The process itself is very disempowering and I felt as though I'd stepped onto the set of some science fiction horror film. I've always thought that all this screening is a form of social control as it does nothing but create huge amounts of fear. I believe there are ways of raising concerns about health without generating extreme fear and the practice of crushing delicate breast tissue. But fear is a wonderful way to groom us into compliance which then silently leads us into accepting treatment we know almost nothing about. Does this seem familiar? It should do, its how governments get to rush through new medical procedures without the full long-term clinical trial outcome. Most people certainly know nothing about the real long term dire consequences of conventional treatment to our health and quality of life. My many conversations with affected women have proved beyond reasonable doubt that we are groomed to stay in ignorance and fear.

It was ascertained I had a tiny lesion behind the nipple so what was all the excitement? So what is the definition of a lesion? Basically abnormal cells and doctors would be at a loss without this widely used term. So it could have been scar tissue from a tumour that had already gone into spontaneous remission. Spontaneous remission is something that the doctors can never explain despite it being a fairly common phenomenon. Tumours can take several years to grow before this detection so what was the hurry for disfiguring surgery? It is a biological fact of life that everyone carries cancer cells and at some point, invariably middle age, there may be signs of tumour cells possibly disappearing all by itself without medical intervention. But I had to remember the body has a powerful ability to encapsulate altered damaged tissue areas indefinitely so again what was the hurry? Making a decision about treatment whilst still reeling from a positive diagnosis could be considered as being unwise and possibly too rash at this very vulnerable time. Receiving a diagnosis takes time to process so any treatment decisions need to be taken after the dust has settled.

What if the lesion was simply calcification or ulceration? Would this be a good reason for such dramatic concern and treatment? The general medical consensus still appears very vague and contradictory. Some are called benign, probably benign, suspicious or malignant but who really makes the definition? Some 'scientists' have proven to be notoriously wrong especially if the bias is leaning towards the pharmaceutical industry intervention. Some surgeons are notorious for just jumping straight in with surgery with no real evidence how a tumour may proceed long term. Even Professor Sir Mike Richards, the NHS's National Cancer Director has used words like 'our considered view' to justify mammography rather than relying on evidenced based studies or medical data that can be actually referenced. This is not to insult the 'experts' but I'd rather not choose my life saving/threatening treatment on some 'considered view'. This is an insult to my intelligence as I don't know how far those subjective considerations have been taken and what the political agendas are, but my personal findings so far are proving these 'considerations' have not been taken far enough. Calcification for instance can take years to develop and as many years to dissipate if the correct balancing measures are taken. This can be a real challenge as calcification is a hardening process so it could take several years to reverse if ever. Tap water can contain large amounts of inorganic calcium so even in addressing dehydration with a view to a cancer diagnosis it's imperative to be drinking pure water or filtered water. As innocuous as tap water seems it could actually do more harm than good especially if fluoride has been added. I occasionally add silica to my filtered water as this maintains a degree of flexibility and softness to the cells which may eventually help to break down these hard calcifications.

An article in a national newspaper observed that the surgeon Ian Paterson allegedly performed many disfiguring operations on women who actually did not have breast cancer. Were these so called cancers found with mammography? If so, were the experts qualified to read the mammography findings? This was followed up by a documentary on TV which also showed how many years it took the NHS to stop Paterson performing his unique disfiguring type of operations. This is abhorrent and it beggars believe that in this day and age, women were allowed to suffer at his hands because he obviously did not work in isolation, he worked with a team. TV's Dispatches programme went on to interview a GP who knew this malpractice was going on but was too afraid to 'whistle blow' in fear of losing his job. In the programme the GP's identity was still hidden. It's strange because when I took a job as a tenancy support worker, it was instilled in us that it was a sack-able offence if we did not 'whistle blow' on malpractices that could affect our vulnerable clients. But it appears this rule does not apply in the NHS.

Studies do show that most people will go on to die naturally of old age without ever showing cancer symptoms. So just because screening can allegedly find cancerous changes, did that mean I and many others had to go on to becoming a full blown cancer patient? Well no and certainly not for me, I have witnessed first hand what a full blown cancer patient goes through and that process is simply not my choice of treatment. It is very difficult and very challenging to start changing core beliefs about the current medical system but I knew I had to if I was to have a long healthy life. An old wise person once said to me that if you want to live long and healthy, stay away from doctors. Deep inside I knew I'd never have another mammogram again. As I and people close to me were still in a state of mild anxiety, I began to consider other options in regard to screening. A friend of mine suggested thermal imaging and recommended a doctor on Harley Street that does offer this non invasive diagnostic method. But screening or testing can be in itself, an exercise of simply looking for symptoms and never the root cause. So I guess it's about who conducts the screening and what to do with the information if a cancer diagnosis proves positive. I certainly did not want to rush into disfiguring/life-negating treatment only to discover it could have been avoided.

I did read about a very sad case locally where the husband after discovering he had prostrate cancer committed suicide. The case was doubly tragic as his wife committed suicide at the same time. I can only imagine the extreme fear this couple felt that the only way out for them was death. I blame the medical profession and the media for touting fear propaganda as it seems cancer is almost being used as the ultimate disempowering weapon of mass destruction.

Whilst writing this chapter I developed a cold which seemed amazing after all the things I do to keep my health in optimum condition. It dawned on me that even with a cold, medicine simply masks the symptoms; anyone will tell you that a cold has to run its course. It was with awareness that I realised the cold had developed because I had been doing too much and thinking too much. I had purchased another investment property, project managed a full scheme of renovation, supported a close friend in hospital with daily visits and also fielded personal attacks from his dysfunctional family after his serious surgery all in the space of two weeks. So I guess it was hardly surprising I developed a heavy cold that basically 'rugby tackled' me to the ground. No amount of medication would have restored me back to health. It may have kept me going longer but medication would have purely suppressed the message which was to stop and replenish myself with relaxation, self care and a few days in bed. It all appears quite simple now.

I'm now seeing cancer almost the same way, it shows its symptoms as in tumours or lesions but do we know or even want to know the real cause of cancer? I fought back angrily when I was asked in Germany to look at the real cause of my diagnosed cancer? I ate healthily, maintained a perfect weight, exercised in moderation so how could I really be the cause of a cancer diagnosis? Eventually I took responsibility for my metabolic breakdown but I stopped giving myself a hard time. I would ensure the correct counselling help were sort that would allow me to make healthy emotional changes. It would have never be easy for me to simply mask the symptoms with surgery, radiation and chemotherapy. I had to make life saving changes, I knew I could not even subject myself to a general anaesthetic in case procedures where done in error or without my consent. Unfortunately, I have no trust in breast surgeons as some of the horror stories I've heard just confirm my suspicions.

Perhaps if we could see screening as wake up calls and if something untoward does show up, we could be simply guided back to restoring personal health naturally. Screening's main objective at the moment may be to get everyone into the 'sick care' management system which could involve several years of expensive treatment that does not ultimately lead to restoration of health. In many cases it does completely the opposite. But as I've already said sickness does generate a lot of revenue especially for professional individuals whose whole life has been dedicated to screening programmes in the medical system. How do you tell someone working in the mammography industry that mammography has possibly been the biggest waste of time at best? At worse mammography could have been turning healthy women into sick women. Archaic screening practices will be doggedly held onto, not because they really believe it does save lives but purely because what else would they do for a job/career and a generous income/pension? I feel we have been brain washing women to conform to this potentially dangerous diagnostic method almost out of habit and misguided loyalty to our precious NHS.

So I watched a TV interview with Dr Eccles who appeared to be the only bona-fide doctor offering infra red screening that had real credibility. The interview was conducted by some mainstream TV breakfast show that can be found on YouTube. I quickly realised this type of screening was definitely for me and it surprises me that more women don't opt for this non-invasive form of health screening. But I guess many are totally unaware that this is available as an alternative. It does cost a few hundred pounds but I'd rather see the results with my own eyes as its happening rather than taking some individual doctor's or pathologists subjective word for it after several weeks.

The day of my of my infra red screening day was possibly one of the hottest days of the year and I had to travel to London on the train without a bra. This would be quite easy in the winter to hide under layers of clothing but not so easy in the summer, add to this the prohibitive use of deodorant and this does not contribute to a comfortable day out, especially in London. I normally use rock salt as a deodorant but just to be on the safe side I abstained as I did not want anything to jeopardise my diagnosis. The consulting rooms in Harley Street were as expected, the usual elegant period building with the added clinical modern extras. I got there early and had to wait awhile but I did not feel nervous this time as I did in the NHS hospital. Finally I was shown into a small clinical back room where I removed my upper garments and sat on a swivel stool. The female trained 'photographer' then took images of my chest from various angles and I then held two ice packs in my hands to see how my parasympathetic system reacted. This involuntary nervous response shows exactly what is going on. The images did show some orange colour initially but then turned blue after the ice-pack had been held for a few minutes. This is good as cancer cells always show red (inflamed) even after the ice-test.

My screening concluded with a consultation with Dr Eccles who evaluated the findings. It was not too scary as my scans did show some vascular activity that he advised monitoring with check ups that were not dissimilar to dental check ups. He complimented me on my adherence to the Budwig protocol and the elimination of sugar from my diet so it was good to have that reassurance. But I also felt slightly flat as screening can create a crescendo of expectation that fizzles out to nothing. Infra red screening is expensive at the moment so I would have to seriously save hard for this type of screening in the future.

Again thermal imaging can be another area where professionals can pull you off track as it was suggested that if the vascular activity did not improve, a new nutritional protocol could be introduced. This of course would involve considerable monetary expense. So I had to ask myself 'where does it stop?' There are as many different dietary approaches as there are religions and I could not afford mentally or financially to hop from one to another. I had found a protocol that worked for me and from my understanding so far, cancer recovery was not simply about nutrition as nutrition is just another facet of recovery.

There is an excellent documentary film now out called The Promise, it uncovers many hidden truths about mammography and goes on to explain the virtues of thermal imaging. I would recommend every woman to watch it as it allows each and everyone of us to make informed decisions on how to handle screening. I believe having this knowledge to be a matter of life or death.

On the subject of screening I feel it would be very beneficial to measure blood sugar or have a live blood test before invasive screening methods are introduced. I watched an interview with Professor Thomas Seyfried who believes cancer is a metabolic disorder. He goes on to say sugar does contribute towards dysfunctional mitochondria. So perhaps testing blood sugar first and encouraging patients to reduce sugar may prevent full blown cancer or at the very least, less aggressive treatment to treat it. If I'd been tested for blood sugar first and it had bordered on a potential danger line I would have taken responsibility for getting it back on track, thereby reducing my chances of getting a full blown cancer diagnosis, which would inevitably led on to a less gruelling treatment plan.

If I 'buy' the metabolic disorder theory that would mean I'd have to ultimately reject the gene theory as fraudulent. But again huge amounts of money are being spent on developing tests that substantiates the inherited 'faulty' gene story. These tests carry patents which can be extremely lucrative for the pharmaceutical industry that manufactures them.

So I had to grow up, take responsibility and question everything. Sitting there in a veil of tears with a doctor or nurse patting my hand saying 'there, there we'll sort it for you' is simply not good enough. They are not gods and it is my body. The health system should be empowering us to take responsibility towards life saving changes. The health system appears broken and overloaded in some areas. But we could be a lot healthier as nation if only we had real choices and knew what to do what to do with those choices.

Non invasive screening could come with choices. Natural healthcare options could include in-depth education as to how the body works regarding nutrition, lifestyle choices and ultimately the damaging effects of stress. So rather than scaring us into taking a one track treatment plan, educate us on how to help ourselves but I guess that wouldn't be very profitable for the medical/pharmaceutical industry? Remember, wherever there is a risk, there should always be choices and alternative options to at least consider.

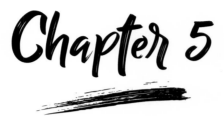

Chapter 5

BELIEFS

You, the reader, may have gathered by now that I am very curious and inquisitive by nature but also an avid real fact finder. This may have saved my life because I've always refused to take any one person's word for anything regarding my health; this also includes advice from some of the so called medical professionals. When someone first suggested that I looked at my own personal beliefs, I wondered what that could possibly have to do with my diagnosed cancer. I had already come to the conclusion that the state of conventional cancer treatments were simply like 'shots in the dark' for many. But what if my diagnosis was wrong? The hospital I attended has one of the worse reputations in the country. The pathology department, at the time my biopsies were taken, were under investigation for using old diagnosing equipment which included pH testing and the time spent 'fixing' which varied on which day of the week the biopsies were taken. This may give false positives. The NHS has also done a sort of U-turn on mammography regarding its benefits and pitfalls, so it's hardly surprising that some of us have deep doubts about the reliability of these so called medical professionals diagnostic opinions.

Taking on an unreliable diagnosis is very dangerous which brings me back to my own beliefs. Did I really believe the diagnosis and the possible prognosis? The diagnosis which I now liken to a witch doctors curse may have already been cast. But was I really going to wear this diagnosis mantle like a real cancer victim or was I to throw the mantle to the ground and stamp on it? Belief is very powerful because refusing to believe a cancer diagnosis could sometimes be mistaken as denial. For at least three to four months I behaved and acted like a cancer victim which could had developed into a self fulfilling prophesy if I hadn't have gone to Germany. In Germany I was taught to examine all my different beliefs and make a start on cultivating a healthier mindset. This was to prove very liberating as that freed up my mind to see recovery and healing as a distinct possibility. It was Einstein who famously said "we cannot solve our problems with the same thinking we used when we created them". So if I created the alleged cancer in my body which I believe to be from acute fear and anxiety, recovery and healing could not possibly come from the same mindset.

A colleague from work told me that his close friend had been diagnosed with ovarian cancer and after a course of intense treatments the cancer had come back. The junior doctor had pulled the husband to one side in a hospital corridor and said "that where cancer is concerned we are pissing in the wind". Not what you'd really want to hear from a medical professional. This just confirmed all my suspicions and I was glad that I had not gone down this one dimensional route of NHS treatment. My beliefs told me attacking and blasting my body with conventional treatment would not cure me in the long term. It appeared to be a short term solution to a long term problem. My long term problem was the incapacity to live well and this was evident by the series of misguided decisions I had made along the way. For me to be well in the long term I had to admit that I had caused the majority of my problems and to take full responsibility for them.

Yes I do agree that some conventional treatments do appear to cure cancers but according to Macmillan – one in every three woman will see their breast cancer return. So does that prove tumours are but symptoms and not the cancer itself? Many women that I speak to who have been given the all clear after a course of cancer treatment tell me that feel they're a ticking time bomb, just waiting for it to rear its ugly head again. That's a pretty scary place to be and it's not how many people would choose to live their lives. Maybe the only thing that's ugly is entertaining these thoughts that cancer is coming back to get us. But the media and medical profession would have us believe that cancer will come back to get us which is why even the most intelligent people continue to live in fear. So as most people 'believe' the cancer will come back, I now know how powerful beliefs can be. Whilst it good to recognise we're not infallible, expecting to randomly die at any time is very soul destroying. To expect allopathic medicine or any alternative treatments to cure cancer is not enough; I knew I had to take responsibility for my own life. Eliminating stress became a priority along with adopting a good nutrition plan.

But where did beliefs and genes fit into all this? My mother died of cancer relatively young, so did it naturally follow suit that I would die young too? If I really bought this old story about genes, why bother being born at all? I attempted to think back to when I was pregnant with my daughter, if a gene test had been available to show that she carried cancer genes, morbid obesity genes, heart defect genes etc. etc. would I have had her aborted rather than letting her live a life that would have invariably turned into hell on earth? I don't know... all I know is that life cannot be that cruel. I now believe we do carry a genetic blueprint from our parents but that doesn't mean all diseases and ailments automatically and actually manifest themselves without our help. I remember a client once telling me that his grandfather and his dad died at fifty with a heart condition and he had convinced himself he would die too at fifty. But how much is down to genes and how much is down to beliefs and programming?

According to a wonderful man called Doctor Bruce Lipton who believes genes are controlled by perception and thoughts, has proved genes can be changed. Only five percent of people born have genetic defects, the other ninety five percent got here perfectly healthy. We can 'learn' to be sick through repetitive programming. He went to share a story that a child had been adopted into a family who had suffered from cancer and yes you guessed it right, that adopted child with completely separate genes also developed cancer when older. A coincidence or a learnt behaviour of beliefs? This made me realise that I had more influence on my health and healing than the medical profession would have me believe. So when the consultant initially asked me "is there cancer in the family" he wanted to make me a victim of hereditary as well as a cancer victim. Well I was just sick of being a victim especially by genetic determinism. I could have used this 'genetic' assumption to enable me to disconnect from my own personal responsibility and hand myself over on a plate to the gods of medicine and the NHS. I could have justified bad living and eating habits with the apathy that I was going to die anyway. I realised more than ever before I needed to believe that my body has its own innate power to recover.

With constant radio jingles and advertising campaigns funded by cancer charities telling us to morbidly look for symptoms at every turn, are we being brainwashed to expect cancer as inevitable part of life? Everywhere I look I see the word cancer from billboards to nice little pink pens being offered at extortionate prices at check outs under the guise of collecting funds for research. It's sometimes called 'raising awareness' by the medical and government authorities but I call it upping the ante of fear. This perverse insidious fear over a period of years can bring on the symptoms of cancer simply because we 'believe' we're going to get cancer anyway. Is the fear built on fact? No, it's built on unreliable statistics and hype. I've come to believe fear is nearly always based on the 'what ifs'. If someone is repeatedly and sublimely told 'one in two' will get cancer, is that a fact or a supposition? But what ever it is the subconscious mind may take it on board which may lead to the development of cancer eventually.

One example that came to light of other people's beliefs was a study in North Carolina, USA, regarding children on the drug Ritalin; over half of the children did not actually have Attention Deficiency Disorder. But the parents had been taught to believe their children actually had ADD and to encourage their children to take the dangerous prescribed medicine. The medical industry are almost hell-bent on making us believe we have a 'disorder, condition or virus' so they can come up with a money making drug that has no real clinical evidence of proof it really works.

Recently on a local BBC radio station I heard how a woman heroically 'overcame' breast cancer with all the barbaric usual conventional treatment. She went on to say that her oncologist had been brilliant but was not into nutrition and had little regard for it. That amazed me because if we were to liken the body to a machine like a car, imagine taking your broken down car to a mechanic and the mechanic said "I don't care what fuel you put in this car just let me fix the broken part." But what if the wrong fuel had contributed to the broken part? "No I'm still not bothered with the type of fuel" replied the mechanic. Would you walk away? Because I had been advised in Germany that if anyone in the medical profession claims nutrition is irrelevant to getting well, I was told to find the door and run like hell. But it does prove that this woman had the utmost belief in her oncologist and she got well. Was it her beliefs or her oncologist?

Medicine does indeed do miracles but it is mostly limited to trauma – Doctor Bruce Lipton

So what was my dominant belief about cancer? I had been programmed to believe that I was a victim with no control. My message throughout childhood was that doctors were the authority on health even though they continued to practise the outdated Newtonian gene theory. So was I really a victim of bodily forces beyond my ability to control? No, I came to believe my body always works towards health if I support it with the right tools. Newtonian gene theory is very antiquated, even more so with the emergence of new research into epigenetics which simply turns the gene theory on its head. Most doctors today will still continue to believe the Newtonian gene theory because it is very convenient and easy for the medical industry and its profits. I have to remember that the definition of a theory may be scientific or even belong to a non scientific discipline or simply have no discipline at all.

My job was now to rewire subconscious thoughts that had negatively impacted on my cells and maybe my alleged cancer would diminish never to recur. Fear was my number one subconscious thought; if I could eliminate fear maybe I'd be okay. Genes do not have the power to control my cells, but my thoughts did. I now believe genes could have the potential to set cancer in motion but it was not the root cause of my cancer diagnosis.

I learnt the environment activates genes and my cells environment is the blood. So the toxic chemicals released by my brain because of fear and anxiety create a toxic flow of negativity directly discharged into the blood. Coupled with other toxins and trauma, I knew this was all associated with my alleged cancer diagnosis. As the live blood test in Germany showed, my blood cells were all clumped together like a sticky stack of coins when they should have been free floating and full of oxygen. My blood (environment) was toxic and that had resulted from constant anxiety and negativity.

Medical institutions appear to operate on fear and anxiety as I have witnessed time and time again, always morbidly looking for symptoms that are sometimes not even there, thus creating conditions that most people are desperately trying to avoid. The scary thing is that the funding and regulatory elements of this medical system know that within each of us is the power to heal. A proven fact is that a third of all healing is due to the placebo effect, in other words the powerful mind has in fact healed the body. Clinical trials do indeed show healing may take place purely by taking a placebo, so how do they explain this? Well not in any terms that the layman can understand. Pharmaceuticals do not want us to know this information, as their whole ethos is based on profit and long term use of drugs. The lady on the radio went on to say after all that harrowing treatment she'd probably be on drugs for up to ten years. These drugs like Tamoxifen have the potential to create cancer according to the World Health Organisation! Profits are of course, incredibly important for any business but not at the expense of people's lives and ignorance.

I came to believe cancer is not the enemy and cancer symptoms are not the enemy either, they are simply 'red flags'. My cancer diagnosis was a strong message, a message to stop, slow down; you're off course, change track now or die. Why shoot the messenger with barbaric treatment? My job was to listen and identify what the message was telling me and it was telling me to let go of fear and negativity. So even though I'd been on this Budwig protocol for a while it wasn't simply about the food I ate, it was about what thoughts I choose to run through my brain on a regular basis. I have to admit my mind was still full of mental clutter and negativity. Guilt and shame was two of the main offenders which at times became very immobilising. I could sense the stagnation of thoughts still in my body. I felt guilty because I still felt fearful and fearful that I still felt guilty. The shame came from realising how many terrible mistakes I had actually made over the years and still not quite having the real resolve and capacity to get over it.

The fear of not following my new regime to the letter held me in a vice like grip. An ingested atom of sugar or cooked fat sent my psyche into a spin believing my body would pull the plug and send me into an early grave. So mentally I was like the others who had had conventional treatment as I also still felt like a ticking time bomb. Even though I appeared to be in optimum physical health, my head was still in toxic overload. I simply did not believe my body would ever support me again. Getting optimistic results from a thermal scan in London did not alleviate my fears as alternative practitioners appear to also plant seeds of fear. Well meaning but ignorant statements like "oh we don't advocate the Budwig protocol, its too much diary; you should be doing it this way". These practitioners will not listen when I say the diary component has been turned into a lipoprotein, but almost covertly the guilt and fear gets instilled again because I'm possibly being told that I'm doing it all wrong... again.

Sometimes, I wanted to scream that it was my carcinogenic thoughts that caused my diagnosis not an innocent splash of skimmed milk in my one and only cup of tea of the day.

Nutrition is important but the advice varies so much, I had to be strong in the belief that my chosen protocol would work for me based on the evidence. Days leading up to a screening appointment can bring on all kinds of anxiety that affect the psyche along with the corresponding ailments. Terminologies like monitoring or watching symptoms like a hawk are quite common in all screening/diagnostic protocols and can also be precursors to fear. A good healthy productive life does not run on fear it runs on hope and optimism. I see many people living on a knife edge waiting for hospital results. Perhaps I could take the longer view, instead of monitoring physical symptoms, how about monitoring the fear that pushes its way past joy and courage on a daily basis? Or I could practise being 'hawk like' into how many negative situations I can find myself in. Instead of a swear box, how about a negativity box? If I find that box is filling up faster than a dam in a monsoon season, perhaps its time to realise that it is exactly these kinds of thoughts and situations that may eventually lead to the abnormal cell growth that creates a positive cancer diagnosis all over again.

Joy and courage were not regular emotions for me so this would take time for me to cultivate and to experience them as normal. Time is all I have so surely I could practise simple emotions like gratitude that can lead into joy. Fear and negativity seemed to be always looking for a way back in and this never felt so prevalent after experiencing some success in the early days. But I was not going to give up as I knew I had to build a bank of positive thoughts to draw on and that meant making deposits of gratitude and joy on a daily basis even when I didn't feel like it. Sometimes the fear fought back with a vengeance and I realised this was my real enemy and not the cancer. Adopting a positive attitude certainly wasn't easy and my good intentions could disappear very quickly but I knew it would be more beneficial to put extra effort into this side of recovery than anything physical. I knew my mind had a powerful role to play in my healing.

A study was done where simply walking through your GP's door was sometimes enough to generate recovery on a simple illness. The mind only does this because of a belief in the doctor's authority on recovery. This was not my particular set of beliefs so it was imperative that I not be bullied or intimidated into taking treatments that I had serious doubts or reservations about. This is why I took the time to consider options and really review various treatments before coming to decision about my own plan of recovery. I learnt to research facts not opinions and I'm continuing to learn the difference. If it cannot be verified, it's an opinion and not a fact. Talking with many people I came to the conclusion that when it comes to health most people are either lazy or searching for a short cut. Nutritional law may certainly hold some of the keys to the resolution of disease but it took time and due diligence to really research what would work for me in the long haul.

The body is not a machine, like a clock for instance where the back is taken off and a defunct part is replaced. We are whole beings and everything is connected, chopping off a breast would not solve my problem.

Throughout history cancer appears to be as confusing as the definition of God. There are about as many authorities on cancer as there is on God and religion. Obviously each authority believes their way is the only way. This was another reason why I would choose my future diagnostic methods and subsequent treatments very carefully indeed. So while surgery and a blast of chemo sees some people bouncing back is amazing but when I took a closer look, I saw that person's disposition, character and determination was what really made them bounce back. They appear to carry a fixed idea that nothing will prevent them from living. This strong self belief may have positioned their bodies to strive for health no matter what; they believed they would get well and they did get well with this particular set of tools. But if reservations are carried about this allopathic route and doubts are entertained, like I had, it would be almost certain this treatment would fail and I would inevitably die.

Taking another route is not about denial, it was about embracing my own personal beliefs about healing. It was about making life altering decisions for the first time ever and this was very scary. I knew it would require every atom of courage possessed. Belief is powerful, suggestion is also powerful. When it was suggested I had cancer, my regular periods simply stopped while my mind processed the information. A coincidence? I think not, that word 'cancer' shut down my body into a state of limbo because I believe having periods to contend with as well would have jeopardised my thoughts and sanity about recovery. As I mentioned before whether it's a doctor or a witch doctor who casts that first suggestion/curse of cancer, like mud it sticks and this can be very difficult to wash off.

I was twelve years old when President Nixon declared the war on cancer. It was not something to really take on board at that age but the message was subliminal, fight cancer and fight cancer like the ultimate enemy. That's a powerful suggestion which over time can cause a belief that cancer is to be aggressively fought no matter what. My understanding is that cancer cells are very intelligent and should I choose to fight them, they'll fight back so I'm really fighting myself. The funerals I have recently attended have proved the more aggressively cancer is fought, the more it fights back. The alleged detected cancer cells were part of me and even though I couldn't put into words why I refused the surgery, proposed radiation and possible amputation, I just knew intuitively that the proposed violent attack on my body was not the answer. I believe cancer is not random, it just didn't slip in my body whilst sleeping from an alien place, I created it. So if I could create cancer surely my intelligent body could create healing.

But did I believe I had the power for healing? Well initially the answer was no. The conventional medical establishment had told me my body had let me down and was now on a collision course for possible death and at the very least destruction. They would help the destruction along its way with the invasive surgery and the burning radiation. It felt like a punishment for 'catching' cancer. I did ask the consultant what had caused the cancer and he told me nobody knows... In that moment I felt utterly powerless and very angry. At this point it would have been easy to say yes to the proposed treatment. Anger coupled with this powerlessness made me want to viciously attack this alien cancer and rip it out of my body. But deep down inside I knew the diagnosis was a catalyst for change. I did not know how change would be implemented but change became the goal. Freeing myself from the conventional treatment made me feel almost euphoric because I anticipated things could only get better not worse.

How could I change me and my beliefs? Going to Germany for a cancer education was a real challenge because it meant I had to suspend my beliefs or learnt collection of subjective thoughts and open my mind to the possibilities that I could support my body to heal naturally. One deep seated belief that I had nurtured is that is was incredibly selfish to put myself first. I remember my mum telling me I was in fact a true member of my father's family because I was selfish, I guess I was about seven years old at the time possibly begging for some toy or treat. Christian teachings also featured large in my life which I took on board as 'put everyone else first' or you will be considered selfish. This transpired into helping others whilst pushing myself to the bottom of the proverbial pile. But I believe now that if I had have put my needs first instead of piously helping others, cancer may not have been diagnosed. My victim mentality ran deep which also resulted in deep resentments and I now know this can have such a detrimental effect on health. Louise Hay, the controversial healer claims resentments are cancer's number one offender.

But how could I re-programme old beliefs and really dissect fact from fiction. Did I have the resources to access scientific evidence and if I did, did I have the intellect to understand it? Then would I have the courage and tenacity to put into practice what I'd learnt or would I continue to feel intimidated by health care professionals who look at me with disbelief when I mention what route I'm taking. It ultimately came down to how badly I wanted to live and to disregard what others thought about my unorthodox healing methods.

As I had done some soul searching previously whilst on a 12 Step programme, I was no stranger to assessing where my character assets and defects lie. So while I could adhere to the physical side of recovery, could I grasp the emotional and spiritual healing that had to be undertaken in order to recover? Well I had to if I were to recover and thrive. Note I say thrive and not survive because I didn't want to simply survive, I wanted to thrive abundantly on all levels.

First my attitude had to change; I decided I was no longer a victim but a victor in life. So how does a victor live on a daily basis? I came to believe that a constant repetition of seemingly small things would eventually make all the difference over the long haul. How could I expect the instant gratification of recovery after only spending five weeks in Germany grasping the basics? The diagnosis had taken years to manifest itself and this could not be reversed with a few months of healthy eating and supplements. The tools I chose for healing had to be embraced for life but I also knew I would not see immediate effects. Choosing not to eat sugar did not have an immediate positive effect on my body or psyche but after two years the positive effects can be seen and felt. Learning to meditate was another area in which the positive effects are not felt straight away but it finally dawned on me that meditation has a powerful accumulate affect. Meditation is fairly easy to do and it very easy not to do, so the choice was mine. Friends often told me that they were amazed by my will power and self discipline but they only saw the accumulative results.

Exercise is also very important in overall health and healing and luckily I have a dog which needs walking every day. But to accelerate my lymphatic drainage I rebound everyday on a mini trampoline, is it hard work? No not really, I jump for about seven or eight minutes to my favourite disco music but if I add that up over the days, months and years, that an awful lot of lymphatic drainage.

Like exercise or diets it's not the big dramatic gestures that matter, it's the little things than gently chip away at old stories, patterns and beliefs and that can change lives. I chose to take responsibility and work towards health on a daily basis. I could either move forward or slide back; I knew I could not tread water for ever. The choices made about my own personal beliefs would be the decision between my life and death. So was I to become a victor or victim? A victor of course.

Chapter 6

NO 'MAGIC BULLET' BUT MANY HEALING PROTOCOLS

I see on almost a daily basis alleged breakthroughs in fighting cancer in both the allopathic and alternative routes but I also know this will never be the true whole story. The only choice I had was to research everything I could to do with cancer and fortunately the internet can make this quite an easy pursuit. But care and caution has to be taken with internet research as it's not always monitored and backed up with factual evidence. I prefer books and papers that can give specific reference to trials and documents that support a particular plan or method of healing.

The whole objective was to find and create a plan of recovery that would work for me on a very deep personal level. I remember a dear friend whose wife had suffered dreadfully with conventional treatment demanding me to explain if other treatments were available, why doctors allowed patients to suffer. I already had the answer but I sensed he was not in the mood to listen at that moment in time as I thought it might antagonise him. The answer to this question hurts and when I understood why doctors were not allowed to tell patients of other less traumatic treatments, it made me cry with incredible sadness. That answer is the 1939 Cancer Act. I could recite it verbatim but I strongly encourage people to study this Act to realise its full implications and the impact on our freedom of choice which ultimately affects our health.

The 1939 Cancer Act is a heinous Act of Parliament which most citizens of Great Britain are totally unaware of but it is precisely this Act that makes it illegal to advertise any kind of alternative cancer treatment in the UK. It gives the 'trusted' NHS and its associated international suppliers (big pharma) an undeserved monopoly on orthodox treatment, almost like a cartel. It does ensure that ineffective, potentially life threatening but incredibly profitable treatments like chemo and radiotherapy can never be challenged, ever.

I could go on but its defeats my journey of positive health but it helps to have an understanding as to why gentler treatments are pushed underground or simply put out of business.

It may be also interesting to look at a doctor's career just to complete the picture of withheld information on gentler alternative therapies. I admit, in the beginning it hurt like hell psychologically to realise the doctor would prescribe a course of treatment he/she knew would not help me much. But not only that, damage me beyond repair. But doctors must use the system and conform to the 1939 Cancer Act or lose his/her job. It does appear complicated but the sooner I understood how a person becomes a doctor, who teaches them and where the information and funding is coming from was a good start to claiming back my own power. In legal terms it becomes easy to understand why doctors cannot talk about the proven uselessness and real hazards of many of these conventional treatments because it does jeopardise a long term customer/patient relationship. I had to bear in mind that the medical profession obviously needs patients as badly as the sick need the hospitals.

Also I was told to bear in mind when a doctor claims to have twenty years experience in a particular field, what it really means is one or two years of training experience with eighteen to nineteen years of repetition. Unlike electricians and other trades responsible for health and safety in the UK, doctors don't have to go back for annual exams to prove they're up to date with current research, trials and safety legislation. Ongoing training and education for doctors appears not to be government funded only industry funded which can be very biased towards pharmaceutical products. We have to remember that pharmaceuticals are big business with an emphasis on profit. Many doctors I know love industry funded 'training/education' as it involves luxury weekends in top hotels with expensive gifts to bring home. Many shareholders and investors also have to be kept happy with good long term returns on investment. I remember an old work colleague bragging about the returns on his GSK shares, claiming it was the only sure investment he could ever bank on because people would always get sick.

Searching for alternative less invasive treatments and recovery methods is fairly easy when one knows where to look but they are not the only answer. There are many other treatments available and unfortunately, for many of us, after being spoilt by 'free' (in monetary terms) national health care, are shocked to realise that many alternative treatments do not come cheap. Many people balked after I told them how much I paid for my cancer education in Germany (it was the cost of a luxury family holiday for 4 for two weeks). My health and well-being will always be paramount whatever the financial cost. Long term, my stay in Germany has paid for itself a thousand fold over but there are other ways. There are some amazing natural practitioners in the UK who can help guide and support the process of healing but this is only something I have since found out after extensive research. It is very important to find a practitioner/therapist that you believe in but equally important is finding one who believes in you and what you are attempting to do. One acupuncturist called me a 'conspiracy theorist', yes you guessed, how could I go again when my three years of research backed with evidence was mocked?

I could list countless therapies in this book and it appears that each and everyone of them has their own avid followers, many who continue to boast robust health years after being given a virtual death sentence. What all successful cancer treatments appear to have in common is total detoxification, a positive change of diet and a mental/spiritual overhaul. I intuitively knew I had to find a way to pull all this stuff together for the long term. This was no instant fix and I remember reading that 'expecting something for nothing is the most popular form of hope for the majority'. I guess not dissimilar to winning the lottery or having a miraculous recovery at Lourdes. But hope is just a beginning. Hope had to be replaced with faith and faith had to jump start some action. As in the Bible James 2:20 'Faith without works is dead'. Initially I wanted instant success or instant healing but I have since learnt it can take several years for a tumour/lesion to be detected. So how could I expect this heal overnight? I couldn't, I had to put in the work and action that would eventually manifest itself into healing.

After choosing the oil protein protocol for my preferred method of a healing diet, it would have been easy to jump to another protocol that sometimes appeared 'better' but a change of diet is only part of the recovery story. So I stuck with it, day after day, month after month until a few years had past. Now this protocol forms the foundation of my 'recovery eating plan' for life. A cancer diagnosis is such a scary thing that not eating sugar and keeping heated fats to an absolute minimum is a small price to pay for health and ongoing recovery. This was only one of my 'magic bullets' and it is achieved in increments on a daily basis.

Eating a healthy plant based diet ensures that once detoxification has taken place this can be maintained by simple supporting procedures. I still like to practice coffee enemas and the occasional colonic irrigation. I've also become a fan of castor oil packing that enables the body to stimulate movement in areas of the body that can become stagnant. I also have a rotating roster of supplements that I choose to take that help support the body during different levels of healing and seasonal changes. Believing that a big breakthrough would come through medical channels was futile for me because I believed the 'cure' was already here.

The most difficult thing for me has been the spiritual and mental overhaul. I have no particular religious denomination even though my background is mainly Christian. It serves no purpose to elaborate on any chosen religious faiths. Only to urge others to use the faith they already have or find something else that works and brings comfort on a daily basis, whatever that might be. Meditation works for me because when I practise it daily, it brings guidance and insights that may be otherwise unrealised. Being still and in the moment whether that is in a city shopping crowd or alone with nature makes me feel peaceful and at one with something. I suspect that something is God as I understand God.

Culling the mental clutter has proven to be the hardest challenge simply because I have been unable or unwilling to let go of things that cause me psychological damage. My mind seems to be always chattering about this that and the other.

Nursing the victim mentality was a bad habit and that's where daily work of 'belief changes' appeared to be a huge struggle. At times it felt like it was set in stone but all it needed was a suspension of one fixed belief and the whole system could crash down like a house of cards that would release me like an inmate from a prison. Letting go of friends who perhaps did not feel good to be around any more was hard as I felt I needed to explain myself. Perhaps by using the old cop out 'it's me not you' would soften the blow as I never wanted to hurt anyone. But I sensed continuing these relationships would do me more damage in the long run. I began by limiting my exposure to certain people so eventually it would become less painful to cut free permanently. A seminar taught me a critical lesson in values which forced me to assess my own personal values. Here are my top three in order of importance – self respect, without this I feel I have nothing and certainly nothing to give others. Self respect is about putting my needs first which gives me the strength and integrity to respect others. My second value is energy, energy to take action and do all the little things that end up meaning so much. There appears to be so much apathy which in turn would kill all my good intentions so having the energy to carry out those good intentions is vital. Finally the third one is emotional intelligence, for me this means not acting like a child when things don't go my way. Or perhaps taking time to think before taking rash action and being honest when attempting to do something negative and justifying my actions with flimsy excuses. Emotional intelligence is about having the courage to speak my truth and knowing when to be silent. I have many other values but these three appear to really resonant with me on a deep level which when practised ensures peace.

So I've discovered there are no magic bullets, only seemingly random pearls of wisdom that have simply appeared over time, which I've now able to string together to form my own beautiful bracelets of healing. If I were to list all the things I have done and things I continue to do would be quite overwhelming in one sitting but what I try to share with others is pick one simple action and build on it daily or weekly. What appears to be an effort in the beginning becomes a good positive habit. Like initially reading food labels in supermarkets, it can be tedious, but only after time, consciously choosing the right foods to consume the benefits will eventually reveal themselves. When I miss a day of meditation which is not often these days, my day can so easily go out of kilter.

It's a series of good habits all linked together that can result into positive health and recovery. I ask myself will it make a difference if I miss a day of good choices. No not really, will it kill me? No not short term at least. But add all those missed days into months and years and yes it has the potential to ultimately destroy my life. I believe picking a healing path and staying on it ninety five percent of the time will guarantee long term recovery. I wouldn't wait for a magical vaccine or cure dreamt up by the medical establishments because I'd be long dead. This world is still light years away from embracing total holistic natural healing that benefits the whole which is why I needed to take personal responsibility for myself immediately.

More care is taken over buying a car or a home than choosing the right treatment route for the body. I was advised to question the doctors and oncologists and if the answers were vague or dismissive, it's really okay to shop around before making a decision. So even if I were to choose the original treatment offered, at least I'd have more knowledge in how to support myself during treatment. Doctors are only human despite all their medical training; they cannot be expected to know everything about recovery if they've only been allowed to legally study one form of treatment.

After all these years of study as a layperson there does not appear to be one single treatment that would ever guarantee a permanent cure and I know this can be very disappointing. The magic for me was to be about addressing all aspects of myself which is not just the body but mind and spirit too. I function better when I allow myself the freedom to come to my own conclusions about almost anything and my treatment was no exception. Dictator type protocols would never work for my character so when people ask me what they can do, its imperative I'm honest. The truth is what works for me will not necessarily work for them because cancer differs from person to person. But I do encourage looking at everything that offers healing potential, then 'cherry picking' a mixture that will work for their beliefs and lifestyle.

Something that saddens me is how quickly people can condemn alternative treatment before they've even given it a chance to work. Many cancer patients will subject themselves to surgery, chemo, radiotherapy and drugs like Tamoxifen for up to ten years, so why would they expect alternative treatment to work any quicker? The positive aspect of alternative treatment is at the very least it does no harm and at the most, it is gently coaxing the body back to health. Unfortunately, many people diagnosed with cancer will choose alternative treatment when orthodox methods have failed. This is turn makes it harder for alternative treatments to work after the body has been mutilated, burnt and drugged into near death. Sometimes it can be too late, so it's not a case of the alternative not working; the orthodox treatment has already done too much damage.

I do pick organic sugar free food by choice but if it's not organic, I let it go and trust my body will take care of any rogue additives or pesticides. Too much energy can be spent fretting about consuming the wrong food. For example spending three to four hours preparing fruit and vegetables for juicing is not really conducive to a happy balanced life and could also be considered quite sad. I consider wholeness is about taking focus off cancer once a sound nutritional food plan has been put into place and living a happy productive life. This may be something many cancer patients may not have had prior to diagnosis so it's important not to replace old stress with the new stress of following a particular protocol.

Having help from a therapist can accelerate healing as I see my own cancer diagnosis as an accumulation of mental overload. So it wasn't simply a physical manifestation of imbalance but a mental one too. Many people I have spoken with about this issue can take objection by claiming they were okay mentally and certainly not mad. I go on to explain that an unresolved trauma can damage the psyche and knock us off balance. It's critical that this damage/knock is restored if one is to live well long term. Emotional healing does eventually manifest as physical healing.

The body has its own integrity and any illness is often a sign of a natural imbalance. I genuinely believe my cancer diagnosis was a physical message to which I had to listen to then make the inner adjustment. If I'd made this adjustments from the outside via conventional treatments, my bodies natural healing powers would have become dulled and may have eventually died. I never wanted to hamper the process with unnecessary possibly brutal treatment. I believe my body works towards healing if I gently support it and let it do what it can do intelligently and naturally.

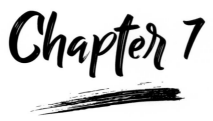

THE CANCER CHARITIES SYNDICATE

This chapter may seem contentious but that is not my aim. These are my own subjective observations which is being purely voiced as a personal opinion. I am aware many libellous actions are being taken against writers of my ilk but my observations are not absolutes only considerations and possibilities.

Some big cancer charities 'undercover' ethics have the potential to disturb me deeply, as I can never really see how generous public donations can go directly into research. Cancer charities, from my own understanding, don't appear to be licensed for tightly controlled research and development. All the alleged new drugs will be ultimately researched and developed by the already rich licensed pharmaceutical companies. Unless of course the charities simply feed these public donations onto the pharmaceutical giants? A good book that could be read a few years ago is 'The Cancer Charities' by Steven Ransom, it is not surprisingly 'unavailable' from anywhere...! Steven's book hurt me on a deep level as it is stated that cancer charities are sometimes part of the problem and not the solution, in his opinion.

So it could appear to be almost like a cartel where nearly everyone involved with the mainstream cancer industries and its subsequent charities appear to be feathering their own nest at our expense and pain. I may be wrong of course and I stand to be corrected with bona-fide evidence if that is the case. I ask myself over and over 'why can't the research show all recovery methods and protocols by financing studies and trials on less invasive treatments?' It's like anything outside of harsh mainstream treatment that can't be patented is branded as quackery even if there is supporting science based evidence and studies. So inevitably, rightly or wrongly I've come to the conclusion that if the treatment can't be patented, which as we know, patented products always generates huge volumes of profit it's not worth bothering with. Unfortunately, if any treatment that is less invasive is having success with healing cancer then the true un-bought scientists behind it may have laboratories trashed with them being bullied or possibly 'dying' into silence. Dr Rife was just one of numerous doctors who had their amazing research and lives crushed by the medical mafia, whoever 'they' are.

This is horrifying and many people simply do not believe it when I give examples of healing treatments being crushed. A friend of mine happened to have a conversation with a security man who worked on an American scheme that ensured all apricot orchards were destroyed. He claimed it was a government order backed by the pharmaceutical giants. The alleged reasoning behind this rather dramatic but bizarre act was that scientific evidence was coming to light that the seed inside the apricot kernel may in fact cure many cancers. So why aren't research charities conducting their own unbiased trials on this amazing natural substance known as vitamin B17? This could be the great new kid on the block? Because apricot kernels are natural and cannot be patented therefore no huge amounts of money can be made from this natural substance? Plus there is evidence out there that does shows B17 works for some people. That's if you can find it now because so many natural papers have been removed from internet searches. So maybe it is purely about profit and eliminating the natural competition?

But much cancer research appears to be nearly always fraudulent with bad clinical trials and bad regulators. A book called Bad Pharma by Ben Goldacre has lots of evidence regarding misleading trials and regulators. Also cancer prevention is not profitable. A friend working for BioCity, the UK's largest bioscience innovation and incubation centre, told me categorically cures were not the aim, it didn't make good business sense. I; state: her words, not mine. Take for instance Cancer Research UK which is the largest independent research organisation in the world and also funds the University College of London Cancer Trial Centre. It transpires that CRUK also receives funding from Big Pharma such as AstraZeneca and

Pfizer. Is this a conflict of interest? This not only shows that trials may be incredibly industry biased but it also may run along the same lines as money laundering with the same money running around the same alleged profitable potentially corrupt loop again and again? Who knows? Its very complex.

There are so many other ways to heal from cancer that does not cost much money, but it appears that no government in the world is willing to fund any natural research. Cancer charities appear to keep the myth going by saying that there is still no cure for cancer but give us a bit more money because we're just around the corner from a break through. Really? They've been saying this for decades. I understand and accept my belief that cancer is a metabolic disorder and there will never be one single magic drug. I believe the reason that no single drug will cure cancer is that cancer is a systematic disorder which affects the whole person and not just a body part.

I'm horrified by all the celebrity endorsements of an alleged single cure. It only fuels my suspicions further that this is simply about raising celebrity profiles paid for by pharmaceuticals. One famous highly paid actress allegedly had a mastectomy after taking a BRAC test. BRAC tests are manufactured by one company who were on the verge of patenting this test and selling it on to the UK as well as American healthcare services. Was this a coincidence? I think not, anything a celebrity appears to endorse, the 'sheep like' mentality of the general public kicks in and like lambs to slaughter, women go and get breasts amputated out of fear generated by clever celebrity marketing. The same celebrity has allegedly now had her ovaries removed just in case she developed ovarian cancer. What ever would she do if it was discovered brain tumours run in the family? Would she go on to have part of her brain removed too? Or how about having all moles removed on the surface of the skin just in case they turned into melanomas. Cutting out and removing is not always the answer unless a tumour is restricting the functioning of a major organ.

Research is now showing academics are being paid by pharmaceutical companies to hype up health scares. Remember the swine flu 'dry-run' pandemic in 2010 that never happened? That generated £6.5bn in the UK alone for the drug company making the anti-viral drug. Most trusted official views can become flawed or skewed simply by the fact that many of them have drug company affiliations. It's this kind of practice that strengthens my resolve to get well naturally and stay well so I never have to fall into this system again.

The salaries of people employed by these charities appear to be well above the national average for the same job in different industries. Some of the 'top dogs' can earn well over a 230-240k a year. I met a young events co-ordinator at a dinner party. She explained that she worked for a fairly unknown local cancer charity but still earns 36k a year, not that much I hear you say. Maybe not now but that was in 2012 in South Derbyshire not London. In 2022 some nurses are still only earning £26,500pa which is astonishing! A glorified party planner and a nurse? Who deserves to be paid more?

If a cure were found and used by the masses, what would happen to all these cancer jobs and the money generated from fund raising? It may not be in the charity or medical/pharma industries interest to find a cure and yet proven recovery and remissions have been around for decades. These unfortunately have been pushed underground only to be vilified by people possibly paid by big pharma to label it as quackery as seen on rather strange website called Quackwatch. The only quackery I see is the barbaric procedures that is still being offered as treatment but not a cure.

Acknowledging real natural recovery exists would mean the end of the 'gravy train', lucrative research programmes and personal glory dreams. Genuine 'triumph over tragedy' stories of real natural long term healing may put a stop to charitable donations by the generous public. But I'm feeling that this is a long way off as the cancer/sickness industry is the biggest business on earth and its not going to go quietly or willingly.

If a closer look is taken at cancer charities you may find some heads of charities are on the pay roll of some pharmaceutical company. These duplicitous people may encourage pressure on the NHS to buy more drugs with a highlighted sob story that may buy coverage for their charity hence more donations. I class it almost like a syndicate and I refuse to be hoodwinked into believing that charitable donations are going to genuine research or trials that actually help the still suffering human being. It is the charities who determine and control the public's perception of cancer; I've often wondered who is actually behind the big advertising campaigns that are always touting fear. My guess is the cancer charities may extract more donations based on fear. The charity called Breakthrough was able to control most breast cancer information in Parliament which is hardly surprising when many health ministers have no real knowledge on health, let alone a biology qualification from school. A health minister that appears to rely on outside information which could be industry biased is not being fair to the public. So the outside information for breast cancer may come from a charity like Breakthrough even though its main sponsor is Zeneca which developed the breast cancer drug Tamoxifen. Tamoxifen was cited as a human carcinogen by the World Health Authority in 2009. It is interesting that there doesn't seem to be a real independent body that actually reviews the work of charities which may have contradictory affiliates. I guess this is what we call trust and 'democracy'?

Politics and cancer are intrinsically linked. I'm still amazed that an American president whilst in office was diagnosed with prostate cancer and went on to have an alternative painless non invasive treatment in Germany which enabled him to live well for almost another twenty years. Did the public hear of this miraculous treatment? The answer is no, the media did not cover this incredible story as we'd all been rushing off to Germany to have treatment that the cancer establishment refers to as quackery. In my opinion Germany appears to have a good range of non-toxic cancer therapies especially hyperthermia treatment which may work for many people including a former president of the USA.

I know cancer charities may invest 'collected donations' into the stock market to raise more revenue but it would also be interesting to see their investment portfolios to ensure the companies are not engaged in the production of carcinogenic products. Pink ribbon logos appear on many products that are actually detrimental to health, like high sugar content candy and sweets, which again highlights profits before people. Charities may even sell partnerships deals to the likes of the big supermarket chains by boasting their 'links with such charities'. This is clever marketing that will invariably increase sales as people do like 'virtue signalling' their public support.

So why don't the government use our taxes or charities use surplus donations to fund education programmes for schools and colleges. Educate young people to take responsibility for their health and hold themselves personally accountable for bodily malfunction that comes from excessive drinking, smoking and over eating? But having personally experienced an education in the UK system, I now realise all my education was geared towards bending to the god of 'authority' and compliance. In other words,'do not question authority' and do as we say as we peddle and support adverts that encourage overindulgence.

The more I understand about cancer by talking with many who have suffered and lost so much, the conventional alleged treatment/cure could be classed as a cruel hoax or false hope? Repetitive misdiagnosis, barbaric treatments and the five year survival will never be a considered a life enhancing solution in my book.

It is hard for me to suggest an alternative charity because cartels are very hard to puncture and expose. There is a charity called Together Against Cancer in Leicester which I deeply respect as offering some real pioneering useful resources and services. When I hear local women have 'ran for life' or some other event to raise funds for big charities, it saddens me when I know how many millions are already in the coffers of these big charities. Genuine small charities like the one mentioned above offer free or reduced price services like counselling, well-being therapies and health educational workshops. Its certainly not squandering its donations on big salaries, fear-malingering marketing and celebrity endorsements.

I've had many charity boxes shook in front of my face whilst walking about towns and cities, which I obviously and publicly decline to donate. The volunteers look askance when I refuse and they sometimes ask why. I try to explain that I will not support an industry that has a seemingly long history of failure. If any new research is shown to be studying the real human condition of maintaining good health and that trials can clearly prove beyond doubt that there is merit in these studies, of course I will donate but that seems light years away as I mentioned before. I have recently discovered that my dad donated monthly for years to Cancer Research UK after my mum died. Did it bring her back or did it help me when I got diagnosed 16 years later? No, but my dad genuinely believed that it all went into research when only 1.7% of possible donations/income goes into cost effective drugs for the public. Source: dyingforacure.org

All I know is that I am healthier than I've ever been and if others could independently research all healing protocols, make informed choices and apply what could work for them naturally, the cancer industry would shrink considerably. "Remember treating disease is incredibly profitable, preventing it is not" according to Dr Robert Sharpe.

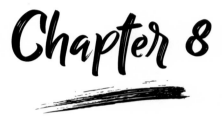

Chapter 8

WHAT NEXT? HERE'S WHAT I DO

After reading about healing and all the different ways to recovery, it can be hard to get started because all protocols can carry the message of hope including the conventional treatments. But some may even contradict themselves especially if newspapers like the Daily Mail are read as the gospel according to the elite controlled media. One day its saying red wine is bad for you, next day the virtues of Revestol found in red wine are being extolled as an anti-cancer agent, the list is endless. Luckily, for me I had made a decision to leave the conventional treatment and the UK within three days of diagnosis and get a real cancer education in Germany. This enabled some of the second guessing and anxiety to be taken away. Unfortunately, I realise many people are unable to do this, not just because of the financial implications but out of a misguided loyalty to their doctors and family. Many people I have talked with often fear what family and friends will say if they start discussing alternative treatment. So they find it easier not to alter the status quo and do what is expected of them. As I mentioned my dad supported me all the way and after that I didn't care what 'other' people thought of my somewhat unorthodox way of responding to my diagnosis. 'Other' people sometimes included doctors and other so called specialists. Many times I chose not to say anything about my choices because I sensed I was being judged a crank and I really did not have the energy or inclination to justify my reasons. I wished I'd known about the 1939 Cancer Act in the beginning. The true implications of conventional medical treatment would have galvanised me to make an even more confident start without the misguided guilt of refusing the NHS treatment.

Having no idea that there was an actual Cancer Act when I left for Germany made me feel like a bit of a traitor for leaving the alleged trusted NHS behind to seek more answers to my dilemma. Because after having a biopsy in the NHS system, a part of me felt as if I now 'belonged' to the medical system. The bruising and puncture wounds that lay protected under my layers of clothing still made me angry but also very scared. By rejecting conventional treatment made me feel that I'd violated national protocol even though my body had been violated by people who worked for the NHS with these very invasive diagnostic tools.

Looking back on my childhood it dawned on me that I'd always felt this way about orthodox medicine. I remember frantically trying to get away, aged four from a polio vaccine. My mother held me down and the doctor was astonished that I was so vehemently opposed to the needle going in. Another time at aged fourteen I managed to somehow avoid the TB/measles jab by joining another queue and fooling the school nurse I'd already had it. Did needles scare me? I'm not sure that was the whole story, I just had an inherent morbid dread of vaccines and toxins. After the birth of my one and only child I had to have an anti-D injection because of my rhesus negative A blood type. I could feel the thick serum in my system for hours afterwards but I was assured this injection was necessary for the safety of future babies. Even though I insisted I was having no more children, I was bullied into having this vaccine which may contain mercury and plasma from a donor's blood. I have since discovered that had the NHS found out my daughter's blood is also Rhesus Negative A I would have had no need for this harmful 'vaccine'/stab in the bottom.

Some of us know intuitively that medicine is not the answer to our imbalances and diseases. It was from this unnamed internal awareness that conventional cancer treatment was refused and I wanted a chance to see if I could reverse the condition naturally. From my understanding of the new biology, it was the environment I needed to change, not only from without but from within. So what did this mean? It meant that I had to grasp that my inner environment had to be my blood. So if my cells, healthy or cancerous live within my blood environment then it made sense to change this inner environment. Many wise new biology scientists liken it with a simple analogy that goes like this: if a cell is liken to a fish in a fish bowl, the water in the bowl being the blood and the fish got sick, would you treat the fish with medication or change the water in the fish bowl? I guess you may choose to do both but it might be an idea to change the water first and see what happened. If you simply medicated the fish and returned the fish to the sick water/environment the fish would eventually die.

So whilst I understood surgery could indeed be very beneficial in some cases it would never solve the long-term problem if the blood remains sick. It was then up to me to create an inner environment that did not play host to cancerous cells.

Live blood tests can be very illuminating as there is no hiding from what it shows in the present moment. It's like a window into the body and once I knew what I was dealing with it empowered me to make the changes that only I could make. Having regular live blood test from a qualified professional during this crucial time helps seeing the visual progress of all the effort made. Live blood tests can also show how well the body is hydrated. Dehydration is a huge issue when dealing with sickness and disease.

So as a foundation to health, hydration is possibly the most important thing I could ever do for myself regardless of the professional opinion of my condition. Dehydration can be a catastrophe for the body resulting in all kinds of degenerative diseases. I have known for years I had not drank enough water, as a young adult I remember drinking loads of cola, even in the middle of the night to quench my thirst. I never even thought to drink water as I did not like the taste of tap water as a child. I believe dehydration began in my early childhood as I was terribly constipated around the age of four. I always wanted juices but mum always said there's plenty of water in the tap if you're thirsty so I remained thirsty as I refused to drink tap water. I knew that I didn't drink enough pure water so I guess over time the effects could have simply compounded themselves into a degenerative condition like cancer during middle age. Whatever treatment route was to be taken I could only give my body time to hydrate if it's to be believed that most chronic degenerative illness begin with dehydration.

A complete hydration programme took me about 3 months of constant daily pure water drinking with a full compliment of adequate amounts of electrolytes, potassium, magnesium, sodium and calcium. I understand without the correct amount of electrolytes the cells are unable to function correctly. I never drink tap water as it sometimes contains fluoride and this substance can cause cancer along with other nasty conditions. I believe fluoride is a ruse regarding dental care as I don't even use conventional toothpaste. If cancer cells were dying off I knew they needed to be removed from my body as quickly as possible to avoid a toxic build-up. Drinking water is the only way I could achieve this successfully or I could soon begin to feel sluggish and bloated.

Coffee enemas were self administered on a daily basis for a year, which then eventually dropped to one or two a week. Enemas are critical in removing any toxic build up from the liver. The liver is responsible for keeping everything free flowing and that included my alleged dead cancer cells. To help this along, I jump daily on a re bounder. This enables the lymphatic system to free up any stagnation that could occur during this process of deep detoxification.

The only way deep detoxification can ever occur in the body is by ensuring all the four points of elimination are unhindered. These are perspiration which is achieved by using rock salt as a deodorant because normal antiperspirants block the pores which is exactly where two lymph glands reside. Next is respiration which for me means remaining calm and breathing deeply especially during meditation. Good exercise like walking, rebounding and ice skating ensures my lungs work to their maximum potential. Regular urination is quite simple by drinking adequate amounts of pure clean water that flushes the body through on a daily basis and last but not least defecation. Opening the bowels regularly and efficiently is crucial to good health or waste backs up like a blocked drain and this would simply be deposited back into the blood stream. This creates all kinds of problems if I remember the fish bowl analogy and why would I want my cells to reside in a dirty clogged environment?

I also took iodine for about four months. A few drops of nascent iodine were added to a glass of water daily and I also added a few drops to my bathing water. If cancer is considered to be a metabolic disorder then it made sense to address the thyroid with iodine support. Apparently iodine used to be added to bread to inhibit mould growth but this has now been replaced with bromide and a few tablespoons of sugar. I occasionally eat bread but never from a supermarket as I've yet to find one that does not contain sugar. An Italian oncologist discovered on dissecting a removed tumour, it contained about seventy two percent fungus. This particular doctor does advocate the use of bicarbonate of soda and iodine. I either bathe daily or at least have a foot bath with a small cup of bicarbonate dissolved in the hot water. This has a very alkalising effect that I even clean my teeth with a pinch of it added to my natural toothpaste. Again fluoride is avoided as much as I can because this may also have a detrimental effect on the pineal gland which is located near the centre of the brain. Fluoride deposits on this gland may contribute to the pathogenesis of Alzheimer's disease. The pineal gland produces melatonin which affects sleep patterns. I consider my sleep to be very healing and restorative so would not do anything to jeopardise this natural regenerating process.

Eating refined sugar of any kind was another priority as sugar allegedly feeds tumours. I was surprised at how much sugar is added to processed food as even savoury items are riddled with sugar. As I mentioned before that oncologists know that sugar feeds cancer because a new chemotherapy that has been recently developed is delivered to the tumour via sugar, which almost makes the sugar like a Trojan horse. My weekly shopping bill is quite low even though I do buy organic where I can. Eliminating processed foods and sugar has saved me an absolute fortune. Only two to three aisles in the supermarket are used now because most confectionery has been eliminated from my diet.

A detoxifying plant based diet will alkalise the body naturally over time. I realised if I continued to regularly eat meat it can be quite taxing on my digestive system so I choose not to eat much meat apart from a little organic chicken at Christmas and perhaps one fillet steak every six weeks or so. Beef contains carsonine which is an antioxidant purported to support cellular rejuvenation. Fish is consumed about once or twice a fortnight if I know its origins but the bulk of my protein comes from the quark mixed with linseed oil which is quite high calorie. But my energy has to come from somewhere. Vegetables and certain fruits are consumed in abundance. I have some interesting recipes for dressings made from hemp oil, garlic, fresh turmeric, freshly cracked black pepper and other ingredients in season.

Regular research is very important so I can keep up to date with all natural methods of healing but also the new conventional treatments that come along. Research should always be approached with an open mind. Nothing can be condemned or condoned unless it has been researched thoroughly. Much is common sense and stuff I've known about for years but it can make a difference in strengthening my intentions for ongoing recovery. There is a magazine that always has its finger on the pulse, which is called 'What The Doctors Don't Tell You', this can sign post to all sorts of further referencing which is bona-fide information. Science should always be progressive and not absolute so there will always be something new to discover.

After studying all this stuff from a balanced perspective I could then consider my treatment options when armed with some evidence based facts. I had to consider that the quantum leap I originally wanted to move from which was alleged sickness to health would be incremental. I finally understood what quantum actually meant. It's a word from particle physics which means that after a period of time, energy will appear at another level with no apparent observation on how it got there. What did that mean for me? As I understood, it meant taking positive steps, however small on a daily basis towards health. Not by big dramatic gestures but tiny little things which on the surface taken individually appear not to make much difference. But compounded over weeks, months and years made massive differences to my state of health. Its called the Tipping Point.

The practice of oil pulling, meditation, rebounding, eliminating sugar and heated fats, and following a plant based diet has made a huge difference to my life, but only in the long term. This meant doing it when I didn't really feel like doing it. It meant doing it when things weren't going well; it meant doing it when I felt down, angry or depressed. It would have been easy not to do it but it was just as easy to continue doing it as a routine is set. Is it hard? No they are simple actions that anyone can take, one day at a time. Friends still think I'm highly disciplined, I think not. It's a habit honed over time that makes it very easy to follow. I want health more than anything in the world, without it nothing has any real meaning for me.

Some people have envied my success with property investing. Am I clever? No not really, I simply had to get out of bed, research and look for properties on the internet and make an effort to see them. Is it difficult making arrangements to view a property and driving to see it? No not really, sometimes tedious but never hard. Did I make offers on everyone? No, I was building my knowledge of areas, price comparable, selling practices, jargon understanding and networking with people in the industry. Then occasionally opportunities would come to buy a property at below market value. My daily routine of going through the motions positioned me to take action quickly because I'd already done work. Some see it as luck; I see it as an opportunity I was preparing for many weeks and months before.

Everyday I prepare my body, mind and spirit for health and I don't always get it right.

I miss meditation because I've overslept. Does that wreck my life? No not immediately but if I never meditated I know I feel the negative effects of general internal chaos over time. My mind and body desires order and meditation helps me achieve order.

Sometimes I start talking with a negative person which is not good for my emotional well-being as it sets me up for a bad start which can slide into a difficult day. This can take me several hours to get back on track but I have to remember whatever I'm feeling does not last forever. Peace, contentment and even euphoria can return within 24 hours quite easily.

A young person who came to view my house laughed when she saw my re bounder, 'how can that possibly make a difference to fitness?' I simply didn't have the inclination to explain that I'd probably dumped 100's of litres of toxic lymphatic fluid out of my system over the years by stimulating the millions of one way valves in the lymphatic system. It benefits my body's immune capacity for fighting any future diseases/viruses and destroying cancer cells. Also rebounding is recommended by NASA as it can be twice as effective as a treadmill. I've discovered to my great sadness that the majority of people simply aren't really interested in long term health and the little incidental things that can make all the difference.

Another thing that was stressed in Germany was not to waste any time or energy explaining to slightly bemused people the route you are endeavouring to take. In these vulnerable first few years of recovery, the psyche can take quite a knock when faced with contempt at the least, going on to utter derision and ridicule at the most. I know this first hand as I have experienced comments like 'what's so special about you that you don't need chemo' to others raising their eyebrows above my head to others like I'm some simple but stupid child. The German philosopher, Arthur Schopenhauer (1788 – 1860) explains it this way, "All truth passes through three stages. First it is ridiculed. Second, it is violently opposed. Third, it is accepted as being self evident." I guess everyone passes through these stages in their own time depending on their agenda. I've experienced my truth on all these stages; obviously the first two can make me feel very uncomfortable. Even more so if the first two are being voiced by what is considered by many as academics or intellectuals.

It occasionally catches me unaware as I sometimes forget about my Germanic advice and go on to passionately explain my personal experiences only to have people totally shut down on me. I then realise I would have got more respect and empathy had I been sporting a partially collapsed body, no hair and real harrowing signs of a personal war against cancer. But unfortunately for these people all they see is a healthy vibrant fit woman and possibly find it hard to believe I had to face this devastating diagnosis but also having the audacity in flatly refusing the orthodox treatment.

If someone tells me a person has recovered from cancer with conventional treatment, I am genuinely pleased for them. They may go on to tell me the person has a real positive attitude and sometimes integrated their conventional treatment with natural protocols that helped pull it all together. Obviously, I would never snort with derision, how could I? Because it worked for them and is exactly the right treatment for them. I do have a true respect for their beliefs, courage and tenacity to get well no matter what.

There have been times when I've been looking for confirmation that I'm on the right path. I'm perhaps looking for support or anything that might remove the doubts that can be felt during healing and recovery. It's very important to state here that the right people should be sought to support you on the journey. But most importantly I've discovered to my detriment it's wisest to keep your own counsel than consult others that may knock you back. Keeping my own counsel means learning to trust my own intuition and this can be strengthened through meditation and stillness.

Choosing what type of people I spend my time with is of equal importance. I'm not saying anyone who doesn't totally agree with everything I say is dismissed; I just find it easier if I'm honest about my core values. At times I can really feel the energy and momentum of life fade when spending too much time with negative people. At that particular seminar that I've already mentioned we were asked to put our core values in order of importance. Still at the top of my list is self respect and the reason for this is I believe my lack of self respect led me to this cancer diagnosis. Putting myself into abusive or derogatory situations is a lack of self respect and I realise it really is okay to walk away.

Energy again is another value that I find is hard to live without. I believe energy begets energy so it's important for me to find people, places and things that inspire my natural energy. I know when passion is missing and life appears difficult energy slips away and apathy takes its place. The long term apathy and eventual depression was a precursor to my diagnosis. So I believe positive physical and mental energy is vital to my longevity.

My third value is emotional intelligence and whilst I realise a whole book could be written on this subject and I believe one has, I'll keep it simple. I feel society places too much emphasis on academic intelligence and this does create unwanted stress. Emotional intelligence for me is now about dignity, responding rather than reacting and self respect. Meditation helps me balance my emotions which in turn enable decisions to be made wisely and responsibly.

One of the most important things that I'm still discovering is how vital a passion for life is regarding healing and recovery. Without this passion I know my body would simply give up and die, albeit slowly. Discovering and developing my personal passion was initially very hard. I'd lost track of what really motivated or excited me so this took a lot of time. I could not focus my life around cancer or even the recovery tools I had chosen, there had to be more. I wanted purpose; purpose to get up in the morning and it began with very small things. Bright sunny mornings walking my beautiful little dog were a reason. Good nourishing food another reason. Spending time with funny articulate friends who accepted me for me was another reason. I realised after pulling myself out of the warmth into a cold stormy Sunday night I'd discovered I had finally got a hobby I was passionate about. Rain lashing against the window screen of my car undeterred me as I made my way to the Nottingham Ice Arena to do a couple of hours of recreational dance. The eagerness to learn more and more is a real passion and this is what my healing is about. By taking the energy out of cancer and redirecting it straight back into the expansiveness of life and things that I enjoy doing.

It may appear that recovery and healing is selfish and indeed it is. But the word selfish gets a bad reputation when taken out of context. One of the reasons I believe I got a cancer diagnosis was because I was depleted on all levels. Too much had been given away to others at the expense of me. Not any more, I have to put my well-being first without exception. I liken it to the safety directions given on a flight about putting your own life jacket on first before trying to assist others. I have to take care of me first, then and only then do I have the capacity to help others. This message is ancient as the metaphor Jesus used in Matthew 15:13-14 'If the blind lead the blind, they both fall into the ditch'. I now realise if I do not have the capabilities to care for myself effectively, how can I possibly care for others?

Chapter 9

CO-DEPENDENCY – A POSSIBLE CONTRIBUTOR?

Co-dependency was not an issue I'd really addressed until three years after the diagnosis. I had done all the other things suggested that may support the body towards healing but I always felt something was missing. After coming back from Germany I guess I'd isolated myself, picking and choosing when to go out and never committing myself to a real intimate relationship. This felt comfortable although ultimately unfulfilling. But I had a lot to do so I kept myself busy with hobbies, the investment properties but also keeping myself fit and well.

However, I did meet someone and it appeared to be a most exciting time. It all happened very quickly once we started dating and within several weeks we were engaged. I was aware this 'falling in love' process is a collapse of personal boundaries. So all my normal protection barriers had been switched off and of course I was blissfully unaware but very contented. I remained unaware, until my boundaries snapped back into place like the proverbial piece of elastic. Some strange behaviours and controlling attributes my new fiancée began to exhibit rang alarm bells within me. Did I listen? No, true to 'co-dependent form', I chose to ignore them despite the painful twang of familiar recognition. We had started to make some very challenging life changes in the form of renovating a dilapidated old property so I naively thought things would get better once we had restored this house and made it our home. They didn't, they got worse. It was then I realised I was possibly still spiritually and emotionally unstable where relationships are concerned. It appeared that I was still incapable of speaking my truth. A normal healthy woman would have walked away from this potentially toxic set up. However, I felt vulnerable after letting someone back into my life and didn't really want to start addressing stuff that needed facing. I now recognise that I sometimes had a pattern of pursuing intimate relationships with unavailable men. Men who appear to eventually be devoid of real emotion or empathy.

I had met my match as he was also a co-dependent but not with me. He had an abnormally close symbiotic relationship with his parents. This was acted out in his many daily telephone calls with his very needy but subtly interrogating father. I felt like I'd gotten engaged to a married man as he always had to 'ring in' to give a verbatim account of all his activity during the day. I had believed autonomy to be natural in middle age but not in this case. This did have a very detrimental affect on our relationship as I began to factor it in as a normal part of our life together and suppressed all my anxiety and insecurities. But underneath it all I felt neglected; this preoccupation to be in enmeshed with his parents was like a compulsion. I felt utterly disappointed that my fiancée was totally unable or unwilling to set any healthy boundaries that may have helped us develop our own fledgling relationship. But I felt even more disappointed in myself as I could see what was happening and I closed my eyes to it all. My ongoing denial soon spiralled back into low self esteem as I became powerless to uphold any healthy priorities and boundaries for myself.

Codependents are often very loyal, remaining in harmful situations too long and I was no different. But I began to lose myself; my once healthy body began to exhibit many ailments from joint problems and sickness to aches, pains and general inflammation on all parts of my body. The healthy regime I'd followed for three years began to slip as I simply did not have the energy to do all the things that once kept me in robust health. I also went through the menopause albeit without any real physical signs but I did become very emotional. Even though we were too old to have children together, I did grieve the loss of not being able to bear children. It felt like a true sign of old age. Without any discussion the wedding was called off and I slipped further into resentment and depression. I sometimes accepted his sexual attention because I felt that I needed his 'love' and affection. But he had nothing to give to me as it had all dwindled away with his past losses, regrets and resentments from his previous marriage and subsequently his messy expensive divorce. The months that followed were harrowing, from cold withdrawal from him to outbursts of rage from me. Our dreams had been well and truly shattered. I knew if I didn't get a hold of myself I would implode and my body would quickly degenerate into a potentially serious illness. Co-dependency is very toxic and I had become a complicit partner in this pseudo-romantic crime.

I knew with or without him, I needed to get well emotionally and spiritually. I wanted to initially save us but I had to accept I could only save myself. Attending a 12 Step Emotions Anonymous group helped initially, to express my feelings of loss, powerlessness and lack of manageability that had now manifested in my life. I applied myself diligently to this programme of recovery but it was too late, we still broke up. The pain and devastation this caused almost crushed the life out of me. I had taken the chance to love and trust again but I had been abandoned by what I thought was my 'forever love' and I couldn't believe life could be that cruel.

It was during the early days of the break-up that I started a new 12 Step meeting called Codependents Anonymous. It was hard because I had no recovery, so nothing to pass on to others. It is suggested that one has at least a year's recovery before starting a meeting but where could I get that recovery? The nearest meeting was probably in London, some 150 miles away. I invested in the CoDA literature and literally prayed for recovery. The meetings had a good core of regular members that came as far as from neighbouring counties. The stories I heard make it perfectly clear these meetings are most definitely needed. Recovery can appear very slow but meetings and connecting with others can indicate healthy progress which in turn, inspires others to continue. Some weeks I went to the meeting full of optimism but sometimes I still felt the despair of losing out to this condition called co-dependency.

The pain of my co-dependency was more intense and longer lasting than the original cancer diagnosis, so here lay my core issue of dysfunction. With a cancer diagnosis I could do something about it, I didn't have to lay back and passively accept a subjective opinion. But co-dependency had involved a significant other that I had no control over and only enhanced my sense of utter powerlessness. I had worked a 12 step programme twenty five years previously with an eating disorder but this co-dependency issue was ten times worse and doubly hard.

Doing a review of my relationships threw up some startling discoveries; I think that I had always been co-dependent and would always attract the same co-dependent dysfunction from others I chose to be with. So my unhealthy way of relating would only attract more of the same. The resulting frustration was the fact that as I aged the co-dependency became more insidious and my denial had deepened. I genuinely believed if I could change myself, everything would be okay again.

The universe obviously had other plans because this process did not fix my relationship. It only prolonged the agony of our break-up. His refusal to accept any part in the break-up allowed him to have the upper hand that simply played with my emotions. Hope became my constant companion, hope that we would eventually be able to have a normal relationship or even a friendship. But the ongoing communication made me feel like an injured mouse that the cat just kept dragging back and playing with for fun. To sever the unhealthy connection I sent an email with some home truths that would hurt him or at the very least stop all communication. It didn't and only then was I able to see the fine line between love and hate. I believe apathy is the opposite to love. So I knew then that we had never experienced real love. So my shameful but unpredictable grieving process finally ended with the feeling of apathy when I thought about him.

As love is all there is, it made sense to go where the real love really resides. I fortunately have great love and support from family and a network of amazing friends. Without them I really don't know where I'd be. Recovery is ongoing and I imagine it will never be complete. But one friend has shown me such unconditional love, care and affection, it has proved I can be the authentic me without pretending to be anything else. I can be happy, sad and everything in between without being condemned or rejected.

Co-dependency has contributed to my difficulties in life and along with the negative emotions of abandonment, fear and resentment which break down my psyche; it has become pretty obvious my body would break down too. I had been living in what Dr Bruce Lipton calls the 'protection mode' for too long which has invariably closed down my capacity for inner growth.

In protection, there is only fear, doubt and mistrust in almost everything. In growth there is love, forgiveness and trust. Some alleged 'love' unions can never nurture the real reason for a relationship, which for me, is to enable the other to become more than they've ever been before. Obviously narcissists, sociopaths and psychopaths never change because the brain's capacity simply isn't there to support a mutually satisfying relationship. Sometimes its so hard to love someone the right way. Also some people don't always want to be loved the way we want to love them.

I am learning to forgive. In personal relationships and business, wires can get crossed which results in knee jerk reactions of animosity. I am cleaning up my act with friends, family and business associates. This is being accomplished with forgiveness, trust and second chances. The feelings afterwards are truly euphoric and liberating. Family relationships are changing, albeit slowly, for the better. I find it easy to make amends with friends as they consistently show compassion after a miscommunication. Whether I have the capacity to fall in love again remained to be seen but I am hoping I have learnt something from these painful experiences. True love and connection would be amazing to experience but do I believe its even possible in this life?

Chapter 10

SO LIFE CONTINUES

What happens now? Start again living life with a new focus and purposeful intention? Unfortunately, this does not happen all the time. I must admit life does continue to throw up interesting and sometimes painful challenges, I often ask who I would have been without this diagnosis? Again I am guessing I may have been a fairly unbalanced person blaming everything and everybody for what went wrong in life. Where would I have been without this initial blow of potential fatality? I believe I'd be taking life for granted. So is my identity still based on 'I was once a cancer victim' mentality? Or has it changed? Yes it has changed; I no longer think about the diagnosis, it feels like it was another life belonging to another person. Could I have got this far in life without this diagnosis and the subsequent choice of treatment? The answer in all honesty has to be no. I'd probably still be scratching a living together, doing whatever jobs I could find, never daring to invest in myself or ventures fearing that it could have resulted in yet another flop like my past experiences. I didn't know that life could be any other than nose to the grindstone working until retirement or death. The diagnosis gave me courage, courage I never knew I had. I am able to do many things without focusing on the outcome all the time. I am now able to do things purely for the fun of it.

Fear and anxiety can still hound me like an annoying prickly bramble around my ankle but nothing like the paralysing stranglehold it once had around my neck. Fear is quite insidious at times, creeping in when I least expect it. Usually it results in a bit of melancholy thought which leads to a slight depression but that depression is normally covering some fear or anxiety. Fear always makes me supersensitive and at times a little paranoid so I always try to start the day with meditation. My favourite is Beethoven's seventh symphony, movement two. I listen to the first three minutes which is apparently a very healing vibration or frequency. Many times it helps, sometimes not. On the days when I see cancer adverts everywhere I feel incredibly hypersensitive and sometimes quite angry. I try and steer clear of mainstream news and other propaganda especially celebrities who have died from cancer or some alleged breakthrough in cancer treatment blazing its headlines across the national tabloids. People sometimes want to talk to me about what they've read but I find it very frustrating because adverts and the press are not giving the full unbiased story. Also people lack the capacity to read between the lines. Tabloids offer the fear narrative which can be very immobilising for many people including myself when I am in a vulnerable place.

Having a hobby, which excites has been very therapeutic as it rests my mind from thinking too much either about work or about ongoing recovery. I can simply be, which ensures I live completely in the moment and when I choose to live in the moment it can be very liberating.

Ice skating became part of my weekly routine. I used to skate for about three years as a child. So starting again after a 40 year gap was a real leap of faith. It was a real luxury skating on a week day in my brand new Italian ice skating boots, meeting like-minded friends and generally keeping fit. I was fortunate to only be a ten minute drive from the Nottingham Ice Arena so it was very easy to make a decision and go when ever I felt the need for physical creative expression.

It took many months of research and listening to others before I could strike the first blow into my own investment business. Property can be both lucrative and risky. I spent a lot of time looking at properties just to get an idea of the comparable prices. Dad became my ultimate mentor because without his building and developing experience I may have felt too scared to take the appropriate action. So without all this combined knowledge I would never know if a property was a good buy or not. Some have called me lucky as I mentioned; I still call it being strategically placed to recognise a good deal that enables a courageous wise decision that leads to action. Fear can creep in insidiously if I think too much about the risks and I think it always will. But remembering how I felt receiving a cancer diagnosis, financial risks pale into insignificance. Utilising the fear into courage is still a concerted effort. Fear renders me useless and courage compels me to move beyond it?

I had lived a fairly unconventional life as I had chosen to live alone with no real desire to couple up. Past relationships and a marriage had been built on compromises and need. What I needed to achieve was an ability to live alone in peace with myself. This took some time as loneliness can be quite overwhelming at times. But loneliness was not going to be an excuse to grab for the first relationship that comes along. I did meet some lovely men but I was endeavouring to practice the art of discernment. After my divorce in 2007 which left me incredibly vulnerable, I made one of my biggest mistakes of my life by involving myself with a man who turned out to be a practising alcoholic.

Anyone who has had the misfortune to fall for an alcoholic will know this has devastating consequences on the psyche. I lived in denial for ages about his drinking, womanising, lies and disappearing acts but felt powerless to remove myself from the awful situation. When reality did eventually dawn on me, the anger and rage had the capacity to destroy me and it nearly did. I once tried anti-depressants in an attempt to mask the anger and emerging insanity but I knew long term, pills would render me incapable of feeling anything. I threw the pills away after a day. It may have been this relationship that could have bought on the symptoms of a cancer diagnosis as I did become traumatised. The prolonged stress I endured for a couple of years may have encouraged my body to possibly and steadily release cortisone that may have caused the suppression of my immune system, death of nerve cells and an inability to kill abnormal cancerous cells. Friends and family barely recognised who had become because I believe I had developed all the characteristics of PTSD. I now understand that I had become a co-dependent but I didn't know how to address this issue at the time so I did go on to find another dysfunctional man to have a relationship with as described in the previous chapter.

This became a turning point so even though I did try to connect with kinder people the co-dependent behaviour had set in as I developed into a control freak trying to hold people back so I'd never get bitten again. The cancer diagnosis shocked me enough to disconnect from these self defeating behaviours but it still took a long time learning how to connect with others in a healthy loving way. Returning to a 12 Step fellowship did help enormously and the ensuing spirituality continues to be one of my most important activities that encourage me to stay well.

Friends are important to me and I always endeavour to make time for a handful of close friends who I meet on a regular basis to do something nice. After the diagnosis I did need to be very careful who I actually spent time with. Negative, energy draining so called friends and acquaintances had to have a limited time exposure to as they did have the capacity to bring me down or bring out my latent people and problem fixing skills. The cancer education I received in Germany taught me, my fixing skills needed to be focused solely on myself.

Time spent by myself is paramount to ongoing emotional stability and well-being. Loneliness is felt from time to time but normally only lasts for less than an hour and these feelings are not to be acted upon by reaching out for unsuitable people who may shore up my temporary feelings of isolation. Learning to live alone has been a revelation as I've discovered how to be a human being rather than a human doing. Life will never be the same again and I don't want it to be either.

The effect of practising the art of living alone in contentment activates the natural law of attraction. Thank goodness I no longer attract desperate, broken needy people.

Developing my spirituality has been of primary importance to my recovery and change in attitude and outlook. I use the principles set out in the 12 steps of Alcoholics Anonymous rather than any organised religion. It means I am free to develop my own concept of a Higher Power, Universal Intelligence or God as you will. Most of the time I am no longer afraid of dying which in turn means I am no longer afraid of living. Fear had held me back from so many things in the past so even though I'm not wildly wading through life trying everything, I now embrace change and new experiences mainly with gusto. Fortunately for most of the time I feel calm and happy with the occasional spikes of agitation. The agitation is normally due to driving my car at peak times which I do try and avoid, the craziness of our government and the insanity around the recent pandemic. Agitation can be positive but only if it propels me forward to take rational action with kindness and acceptance.

My dream is that whoever reads my experience of a cancer diagnosis and my subsequent journey will be inspired to ask even more questions. Then be motivated to seek for all the different answers to healing as it will always be a fascinating and somewhat scary journey of discovery. It is hoped that some time in the near future people can all come together and pool all resources to share with others, others who may be facing this devastating diagnosis alone. It would great to hear about methods that have worked well and others that may have failed. The greatest thing would be uncensored public feedback on protocols that have been taken further to achieve even greater results. If I had to remember anything, it would be the body always works towards healing. I believe my body would never set out to intentionally kill me. But my body needs my consent and support but also the support of the universe which I choose to call God, to assist fully in this process of healing.

Chapter one began in November 2011 with my scary first visit to the doctors surgery. The even scarier mammogram and biopsies took place around Christmas 2011 and what a happy Christmas that was...not! My official diagnosis came on the 12th January 2012 and I was in Germany on the 15th January 2012. I began this book in 2013 and got the first, albeit rough, edition self published mid 2016. I moved from Nottingham to East Anglia in 2018 and I started revising this book in September 2022.

To date I live with my partner of almost six years. Being in a relationship is not easy for me as I feel I lack the basic components for real consistent contentment. And sometimes I feel my expectations are too high which places high demands not only on myself but on others too. I am definitely a free spirit so resist being controlled or contained by the state, the NHS, family and friends at all times. I do abide by the law as do prefer peace so I pick my legal battles wisely. Health and serenity is my priority with only a few colds and sports injuries over the last decade to hamper my consistent good health. I feel fit, strong and fresh despite my years and have never suffered any serious or chronic conditions. My breast is still slightly retracted and its something I live with because it has never changed. The doctor told me over 11 years that I had cancer and needed an amputation. I have never been given the 'all clear' by the NHS but I have to trust that my body supports my life and rise above the morbid speculation of cancer. My mental health did suffer during the 'covid-era' with a touch of agoraphobia. Fear appeared more contagious than a virus and I couldn't bear to see all the terrified eyes behind the masks. I never thought that I would witness loss on such a huge scale from lives, jobs, livelihoods, education, freedom of speech, travel, debate, democracy, banking and the list goes on and on. I have known for a couple of decades that this was coming with the scare of swine flu in 2010 and other pandemics that didn't actually take off. But this did take off and in my life time. I genuinely believed that I would be dead and buried before a virus actually shut down the world and changed it for the worst. I used my time wisely during the 'covid-era' and studied real law which has helped me immensely to stay lawfully free from restrictive legislation. I am incredibly blessed and fortunate to live ten miles from the beautiful Suffolk coastal town of Southwold. I had always wanted to live near the sea and East Anglia has to be the perfect retirement location for me. Gazing at the sea's horizon makes me feel very serene and can be a great leveller. Our home is a modern rural retreat set in a couple of acres of parkland which is great for my ageing Jack Russell and me to potter around in private peace. My adored little dog has always been my constant companion through all the good times and bad. I actually passed my motorcycle test here in Suffolk aged sixty and cruise the Suffolk and Norfolk country lanes on a Honda CB500 motorbike in the summer. Sometimes alone or when I am feeling more courageous, with my bike mad/car mad partner. Riding a motor bike is better here as the population is sparse and the roads are relatively quiet. I still can't believe that I can handle and ride a big bike confidently and safely as people always look astonished that I even have a motor bike. Should two wheels become too much as I get older, my dad and I share an investment vehicle, a stunning Morgan which has been my dream car for over forty years. Suffolk is the ideal place to have one of these compact vintage vehicles. Driving around leafy lanes and picturesque towns and villages feels like I've time travelled back into the 1950's or 60's, oh the good old days. Its been almost eleven years since that diagnosis which feels like a life time ago. Life is a thousand times better than before the diagnosis and the effort has all been worth it to this day.

Above all this is my memoir and musings on a cancer diagnosis, my personal health and life in general. The diagnosis changed me more than I can ever say and life will never be the same again. For that I am eternally grateful.

Anyone mentioned in this memoir are simply my own subjective observations and I do not intend to represent or misrepresent his or her research/work/experience.

Appendix

Books for further reading:

Chemotherapy heals cancer and the world in flat
– Lothar Hirneise http://hirneise.com/

The Field – Lynne McTaggart

Quantum Healing – Deepak Chopra

Bad Pharma – Ben Goldacre
https://www.badscience.net/about-dr-ben-goldacre/

The Emperor of all Maladies – Siddhartha Mukherjee

The Biology of Belief – Bruce Lipton

Mammography Screening – Peter C Gotzsche
https://www.deadlymedicines.dk/about/

The Oil Protein diet – Johanna Budwig
https://budwig-diet.co.uk/

The Secret to Healing Cancer – Dr Tien Sheng Hsu
https://www.facebook.com/DrTienShengHsu/

Fats that heal, fats that kill – Udo Erasmus

Cellular Awakening – Barbara Wren

Our return to the light – Barbara Wren

The slight edge – Jeff Olson

Websites-
www.oilpulling.org
www.gerson.org

Recordings:
Biology of Belief – Bruce Lipton
Latest training – Bruce Lipton

Films & Documentaries:
The Promise – A Nark Angel Production
https://vimeo.com/77088100
Can you trust your surgeon – Dispatches – Channel Four

Lectures:
Benefits of Papimi by Dr. A Bentas –
Germany – January/February 2012
Bad Pharma – Dr Ben Goldacre – Nottingham,
England – November 2012

Courses:
A five week residential course at the 3E Centre near
Stuttgart, Germany to learn the 3E programme of nutrition,
detoxification and mind work. https://3e-centre.com/

PSYCH-K – copyright. To become a PSYCH-K
facilitator to help change beliefs.

Manufactured by Amazon.ca
Acheson, AB